dimension of aerial being . . . This beautiful, moving book is both a gift from and a tribute to its author, a daring, brave, poetic articulation of the transcendence of flight.'

Isabella Tree, author of *Wilding*, *Literary Review*

'A profound, euphoric and courageous book about how to live joyously, and how to meet death . . . breathtaking . . . Her journey is as lyrical and complicated as the sky she describes, and her book is a shimmering parting gift to those still earthbound'
Guardian

'*Skybound* is a soaring gift of a book. A moving meditation on landscapes and the leaving of them, the freedom of travelling beyond our fears and how our journeys between the known and the unknown, the familiar and the unfamiliar can teach us to cherish and see again'
Owen Sheers

'It's early for predictions, but I'm sure Rebecca Loncraine's *Skybound* is going to be one of my books of the year. It's a book that makes you look at the sky and the land with new eyes; that gives you a lift, in more ways than one . . . an extraordinary book . . . a celebration of wind and wings . . . we've lost a huge talent'
Daily Telegraph

'Stunning. Rebecca Loncraine is a beautiful writer and thinker and *Skybound* is so full of life — a love letter to nature and a hymn of love to the parental bond'
Cathy Rentzenbrink, author of
The Last Act of Love and *A Manual for Heartache*

'A valuable contribution . . . . young pilot who will sadly neve . . . . nanual for anything, it's for how . . . . uncertainties . . . I won't soon . . . . ht, on home and family. . . "Lea . . . . ke asking the un . . . . r with joy and the . . . . t the universe

agreed to Loncraine's request, and that in return it asked only that she leave us with this remarkable book'

Mark Vanhoenacker, author of *Skyfaring*, *Spectator*

'If you're looking for beauty, love and courage, read this book'

Nicholas Crane

'Reading *Skybound* is the closest you will come to flying without sprouting wings. It is an astonishingly beautiful book, a record of a life that, although heartbreakingly short, was lived vividly and thrillingly and intensely. We must all strive to do what Rebecca undoubtedly did – honour the miracle of our existence. She has left the world with something brilliant and unique'   Niall Griffiths, author of *Grits*

'A life-affirming memoir'   *Radio Times*

'As thoughtful and insightful as it is courageous and inspiring'

Sunday Express

'As much a biography of the air as it is a deeply moving memoir, this beautiful book transformed the way I see the sky. I learnt so much about how the air behaves, the physics of gliding. And Loncraine's affinity for the birds she observes and flies with shines through this fascinating, lovely book'   James Macdonald Lockhart, author of *Raptor*

'*Skybound* is a profound and exquisitely written witness to the author's flight and fear, wings and woundedness. Then it lifts into something beyond: the beautiful blue brilliance of her mind's sky'

Jay Griffiths, author of *Wild: An Elemental Journey*

'*Skybound* proves that one can soar above the fear of death both literally and in language of unsurpassed beauty . . . the book is about the sheer thrill of being part of the astonishing earth we have in common, written by an extraordinarily sensitive and gifted writer'   *Harvard Review*

'I have never read anything like it. A portrait of a young woman in love with the sky, painted from a palette of courage, honesty and moments of great beauty'   Jim Crumley

SKYBOUND

Rebecca began writing *Skybound* after recovering from breast cancer. She became unwell again in 2015 and died in 2016, just as she was finishing the book. *Skybound* was, and still is, a book about learning to live again: gliding transformed Rebecca's world.

Bird Girl

I feel you are
somehow, somewhere
rising up like a child
from her bed;

like a crane lifted up
over himalayas of grief
on a column of air
by the grace of light

Ben Brice

Rebecca Loncraine

SKYBOUND

A Journey in Flight

PICADOR

First published 2018 by Picador

First published in paperback 2018 by Picador

This edition first published 2019 by Picador
an imprint of Pan Macmillan
20 New Wharf Road, London N1 9RR
Associated companies throughout the world
www.panmacmillan.com

ISBN 978-1-4472-7387-5

To my mum and dad,
Trisha and Tony Loncraine,
with love.

'No bird soars in a calm.'
Wilbur Wright

Contents

PART THREE: THE BLACK MOUNTAINS, WALES &
THE ANNAPURNA RANGE IN THE HIMALAYAS, NEPAL

Prologue

Blackbird

The blackbird perches on the topmost branch of the tree at the end of my garden. It's spring. He trills and whistles, chirrups and flutes, slides up and down a scale of notes, singing out his place in the world.

It's a stormy afternoon and low cloud and thunder roll up the valley towards my back door, where I sit on the step, flecks of rain blowing into the kitchen. I look out across my small garden and see two squabbling thrushes fly through the rain, jackdaws shelter in a weeping willow, hunched black shapes among dripping branches that sigh down to the ground, and wood pigeons perch, cooing down the chimney.

Another blackbird further down the street sings particularly loudly, and I set out in the rain to get a closer look. I reach the tall tree where he bobs and sings. I try to listen – really listen. His voice soars, pitches down, loops back around the same high phrase, speeds up, slows, and pauses, I imagine, to listen. Another blackbird across the road sings from another tree. The two birds take it in turns, sing and listen, call and respond. As my ears slowly attune and my hearing sharpens, I become aware that blackbirds are singing across the whole small town, and out in the field and woods at the back of my street. They sing unselfconsciously, and I feel mute by comparison – a dumb animal embarrassed by her voice, my words clumsy.

I am sheltering under a beech tree that overhangs the road. Droplets fall from the leaves on to my neck and roll down the inside of my jacket.

A woman steps out of her front door. 'Can I help you? Are you lost?'

I've been wandering back and forth in front of her house, notebook open and pen scribbling, staring up at the rain. I smile, apologize; I must look strange. 'I'm writing about blackbirds,' I tell her, realizing just in that moment that this is what I'm doing.

'Oh, my garden is full of them,' she says. 'The place is alive with them,' and I think, Yes, how well put: it is alive with them. Their song is visceral, while my words seem linear and disembodied.

Behind this feeling of muteness looms the task I've set myself, of giving an account of my own experiences up in the sky, in the realm of the birds – experiences which are almost beyond language to me. In setting out to write this story, I feel like it is me who is perched precariously at the top of a waving tree in the middle of a thunderstorm, face lifted upwards, beak open, trying to find my voice. I'm daunted, feel bound to fail, or at best to fall far short. 'Language does not express the dumb feelings of the mind,' wrote Richard Jefferies, 'any more than a flower can speak.' And yet there's something about survival in this searching for a voice, and something exhilarating about being on the edge of the expressible, so I have no choice but to make the attempt.

Part One

The Black Mountains, Wales

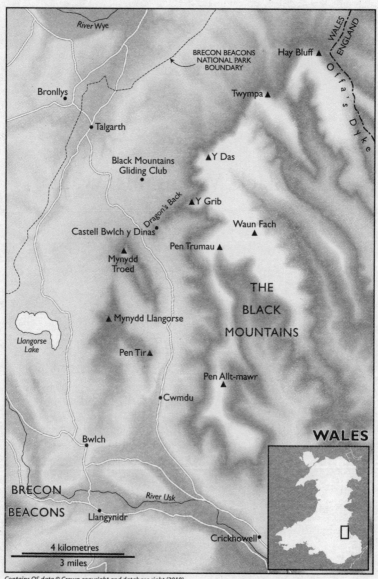

Contains OS data © Crown copyright and database right (2018)

Chapter One

Take Off

The ground falls away beneath me at seventy miles per hour and I am swallowed by the sky. The air howls and I glance down at a panel of dials with twitching needles. I don't know what they mean, but I watch them anyway. I'm sitting in the front seat of a glider for the first time. The clear canopy, only inches from my head, is like a bubble over me; I have a 300-degree view and any sense of confinement inside the tiny cramped cockpit has melted away; I'm jutting out into the air, like a carved wooden figure on the prow of a ship pushing forward into the elements: I am right up against the sky. We are attached by a sixty-metre rope to a small plane that's towing us up from the airfield in the Black Mountains of Wales. We are being towed up into the air because this aircraft has no engine, no internal source of power whatsoever. Bo, an experienced pilot and instructor, is flying the glider from a seat behind me.

I stare in astonishment at the shrinking ground below. Bo tells me he will release us from the towplane. I hear a clunk, feel a jolt, the towplane continues forward, but we slow down and tip to the right. The horizon is at thirty degrees in my view. The towplane disappears and we're left here, suspended in the air, 1,500 feet above the ground, with no source of power.

But the nervousness that beat through my body ten minutes ago, before I stepped into this strange engineless plane, has fallen away with the ground. I left it down there. I feel calm, transfixed by what I can see and where I find myself. This hot spring day in late April, the sky is almost cloudless; it's a big blue empty space, a nothingness above the ground.

The landscape below is clear and strange. Curved fields edged with hedges roll out in every direction from the base of the hills, spreading down valleys to meet rivers and roads that twist and wind as they move from one stony scribble of a village to another.

We move in wide circles, then head straight and level, then tip one way with a wing pointing down at the ground for a moment, then tip the other way. We climb and climb. The ground continues to shrink, and the human world has almost disappeared by the time we reach 6,000 feet. It's as though we've moved back in time while climbing in altitude; I can't see any cars moving through the land-scape, there are no tractors ploughing fields, no telegraph poles or power lines.

The shape of the Black Mountains is clear now, and I get an aerial overview of this body of hills for the first time. I thought I knew them, but now I realize that my knowing was on one narrow scale; as soon as I'm above the ground, I'm lost.

In the distance, the dark silhouette of the larger Brecon Beacons looks like a painted backdrop in an old Western movie. The top of Pen y Fan, the highest peak of the Beacons, points up into the hazy sky.

Below me, Llangorse Lake is a slate-grey curve. Every field is at an odd angle to another, and nothing is square or symmetrical or flat. Instead, everything sweeps up or down or sideways, though any idea of what is a 'side', a 'front' or a 'back' makes no sense from up here. Circling, tipping and weaving, the movement of the aircraft through the sky seems to mirror the rounded shapes of the undulating landscape below.

Looking straight ahead to the horizon, the sky is a watery colour, and, directly above, it's a darker Prussian blue.

I'm shocked to suddenly notice that we're flying directly over my home, the place where I grew up and where I recently returned to live. It's a hill farm, tucked into a long, thin valley that snakes between two hills. I've never seen it like this before, all at once, and for the very first time I can look at its overall shape, its body. I trace the boundaries of the farm with my finger from inside the glider. I see how the land rises up and wraps around it on three sides, so it looks like it's held in the cupped hand of the hill. Beyond the farm, I can see how it sits within the wider landscape, and I've a feeling of rediscovering my familiar world, but from a much larger perspective.

On the ground, I know this terrain almost better than I know my own body, but up here I find it hard to make sense of. I have to re-familiarize myself with it, scanning the land in search of the farmhouse, barns and yard, and the shapes of the road and river that cut down through the middle of the valley. It feels odd, like bumping into some-one you know well in a completely unexpected context.

We descend a few thousand feet, and I'm able to make out the animal tracks that criss-cross the tops of the hills above the farm and which I've walked countless times. In ten minutes, we swoop over terrain that takes me six hours to hike. I'm smiling – a broad, natural smile – and I lean back on to the grey parachute I'm wearing, to look up into the blue. I feel on the edge of something.

We weave down to 1,000 feet above the ground, fields enlarge, familiar hills loom above us once again and we head back towards the airfield. My hands have rested on my thighs throughout the flight. Bo asked me if I would like to take the controls and have a go at flying, but I said no; thanks, but no.

We land, roll along the grass, stop still and tip on to the left wing. Bo opens the canopy and helps me out. I'm still grinning. The flight was about forty-five minutes, but it seemed much longer. Time has stretched and deepened. Gary, another pilot, comes to meet us on a quad bike to tow the glider back to the launch point. He looks at me and smiles. He knows what a first flight can be and there must be something in my face – I'm burning with a sense of uplift.

*

I made the decision to fly an unpowered aircraft at a time when I was sunk under the weight of grief. It was a giant stone in my chest, lying beneath the scar where the tumour was removed. In my mid-thirties, I was exactly one year out of a year of gruelling treatment for breast cancer. I'd lost four stone and my hair was still wiry from the chemotherapy. When I looked in the mirror, I was reminded of a cornered wild creature. I didn't recognize myself. I was still reeling from the shock of the diagnosis and its appalling treatment. In a sense, the ground had already disappeared from beneath me.

The discovery of the lump and the diagnosis was quickly followed by six rounds of chemotherapy over five months, one every three weeks. Every round would leave me bedridden for a week, feeling like a dying animal trying to crawl forward into the opaque half-light at the edge of the living world, before being taken for the next round. The chemo pushed me to the brink of my endurance and far out beyond it. Bald, thin and exhausted, I then underwent invasive surgery and radiotherapy.

During the year of treatment, the rest of my life disintegrated. I separated from my partner, the brightest, kindest and funniest man, but, for reasons beyond our control, we couldn't look after one another. I also left the rented house and the town where I had lived and worked for a decade. Most of my belongings were boxed up and in storage. A voracious reader and scribbler, I had stopped both reading and writing.

In the midst of this crisis, I moved back to the remote

hill farm in the Black Mountains of the Brecon Beacons National Park in Wales, where, from the age of twelve, I had grown up, and where my parents still live. The farm is eighty acres of steep patchwork fields along one side of a horseshoe-shaped valley, with a river running down the middle of it. The old stone farmhouse, with its metre-thick walls and big fireplaces, is at the top of the valley. It's essentially a rocky outcrop of the mountain above, and the wildlife happily inhabits it: swallows nest in the barn, bats roost under the eaves (and in the bathroom, if you leave the window open at night), bumble bees live in the wool fleeces used for insulation in the walls; wagtails, wrens, flycatchers and fiery bobtails nest in holes in the stone-work, wasps nest in the roof and solitary bees creep from beneath the tiles. Several years ago, Mum woke one night to find a hedgehog under her bedside table. The front door is wide open most of the year round and the flagstones on the kitchen floor merge seamlessly with the stone front porch and the yard beyond; there's no real boundary between the house interior and the valley outside. To return to the farm after almost ten years of town-living was to be immersed again in the natural world.

My life had unravelled and I had gone back to what felt like a place to begin again. My loving parents took me in and held me throughout my treatment. First, Mum accompanied me to the hairdressers to have my shoulder-length hair cut off in preparation for chemotherapy. She telephoned the hairdresser in advance to explain the situation and sat next to me as the young woman silently cut the long locks in rough chunks to get it over with quickly. There was no talk of holidays. Both Mum and Dad accompanied me to every chemotherapy session, sitting with hot drinks as the nurse injected litres of bright red liquid into my blood. Each time we left the chemotherapy room, Dad held the door open for Mum and me and thanked the nurse, as though we were leaving a restaurant.

Back at home, Dad managed lambing alone for the first time, leaving Mum free to commit herself utterly to supporting me through my treatment, barely leaving my side throughout the year of hospital appointments. She made endless squash soups, porridge and anything else soft I could eat. She boiled our untreated spring water for me to drink the regulation two litres a day, took my temperature twice a day, keeping an eye out for infections while I had no immune system, and, her greatest achievement, she hid her own pain from me, patiently getting through the long hours in hospital waiting rooms filling in crossword puzzles, as her only child fought to stay alive. After my operation, surfacing from the anaesthetic and afloat on morphine, my immediate thought was that the first person I wanted to see was Mum, so I kept my eyes closed as I was wheeled back to the ward until I heard her voice and knew she was sitting next to me.

At home, when I fell asleep upstairs in my room above the kitchen, I listened to the reassuring voices of Mum and Dad below, muffled through the floorboards and my pillow, and I was sent spinning right back to childhood. The cadences of their voices created a comfortable cave of sound in which to fall asleep. I was so relieved to be back at home, in a place that was precious to me, and where I hoped I could recover.

*

During that first flight, I thought I'd never seen the farm from the perspective of the sky, but later I recall that I have – in a photograph. Throughout my late childhood and adolescence, a photograph, taken from the air, of the farm and the hills surrounding it, was pinned to the noticeboard next to the telephone. It was an old phone, with a yellow spiralling cord, and you had to stand within a few feet of the noticeboard to use it. I spent many hours talking on that phone, often resting my eyes distractedly on that strange image. So, in many ways, this view of my world from above was always just in the corner of my eye. I vaguely knew that Dad had had a few flying lessons locally. He said something about it at the time, but I didn't grasp properly what it was he was talking about and I certainly had no idea he had flown without an engine; I couldn't have imagined how that was possible.

This photograph of the green valley, hills and blue sky, taken at a slight angle 1,000 feet or so above the hilltops, the altitude that soaring buzzards fly, held its position in our lives over many years, slowly bleaching in the light from the window. I don't know what it meant to Dad. A moment lifted out of the sometimes gruelling business of life on the farm, perhaps. Then, a few years ago, it disappeared from the noticeboard. Mum treasures the photographic archive of our lives and has, over the years, organized all the loose photographs into labelled subsections kept in a huge drawer. I think I have no hope of finding the photograph again, but I look through the drawer and, amazed, I find it under a section entitled 'Nature & Oddities'. There's no evidence of the glider in the picture – no wing tip or canopy is in view. Dad must have stuck the camera lens out of the small air vent in the side of the canopy. But, all those years it was pinned to the noticeboard, I half believed, in the way you can hold a daft idea at the back of your mind, that it was taken by a buzzard.

I must have expressed an interest in the photograph because, on my eighteenth birthday, a blue card with a drawing of a glider on the front and the word *Voucher* appeared. I could go to the gliding centre and exchange it for a trip into the sky. I held it in my hand, stared at it and knew for certain that I wouldn't use it.

As a child, I hadn't been afraid of flying, but as I approached adulthood I slowly became more and more fearful. There was always something emotionally raw and heightened about flying for me; perhaps it was some association I made after, 30,000 feet above the Pyrenees in a commercial jet, aged twelve, travelling to Spain on holiday, I discovered the first spots of blood in my knickers while visiting the loo. This shock of redness was so completely at odds with the white plastic washroom – a stark animal secret that must be kept hidden amongst all the technology. Thereafter, my periods, I noticed, would often come on during a flight. Perhaps it was the air pressure (commercial jets can only pressurize to the equivalent of around 8,000 feet, hence swollen feet and the threat of deep vein thrombosis).

For me, flying always had something akin to the hormonal sensitivity of menstruation, and my fear of flying dug deeper until each trip abroad became an ordeal. My palms would drip with sweat, leaving damp patches on my thighs, as I imagined that crucial bolt in the engine working its way loose. Flying over the Atlantic, especially if it was a night flight, I'd think about the sea beneath us, the freezing choppy waters, and the giant squid and devilfish waiting for us to plummet into the icy depths. If it was turbulent, images of crashing would fly through my mind as fast as the plane was travelling, and I'd imagine a horror show of melodramatic and gruesome scenes: women screaming in their seats, men falling to their knees in prayer in the aisle as we dived into the sea. In the end, I resorted to taking anti-anxiety medication.

But I couldn't bring myself to throw out the faded blue flying voucher. It remained in my underwear drawer in my bedroom on the farm for many years. On visits back home, after I'd left, I'd open the drawer to rifle around for a clean pair of knickers and there the voucher would be.

*

Since the end of the treatment, I've been slowly walking myself well. Two hiker friends, Nick and Polly, who know every inch of these hills, have been guiding me through ever longer, steeper walks. At the beginning of the year of recovery, I could barely walk a mile on the flat; now, we hike all day.

During these walks, our conversations wind and meander, unlocked by our steady pace. On one particular hike, Nick told me about his skydiving experiences back in the late 1970s, and about the strange obsession that overtook him then and led to him leaving his job to work at the parachute club, even sleeping under the parachute packing table sometimes. He said it was exhilarating to throw himself at the ground from 12,500 feet and miss, to indulge a suicidal urge, but then dodge it and survive.

'Time alters during a jump,' he told me. 'It slows down and expands. A few seconds in free fall feels like the equivalent of several minutes on the ground.' When you reach terminal velocity in free fall, about 120 miles per hour, he recalled, you no longer have any sensation of falling; you feel like you're being held up by the air, like you're flying. You can twist and move your body about. But, once you reach 3,000 feet, the 'ground rush' begins; the earth hurtles towards you fast and there's an acute sense of urgency to pull the cord to open the parachute.

Hearing Nick talk about his skydiving brought me back to the faded aerial photograph by the telephone and the unused flying voucher. By then, my relationship with fear and risk had totally altered: cancer had stripped away any delusion of safety on the ground. Suddenly, I wanted to face fear head on – to choose it, move towards it, become intimate with it – and, in this choosing, I hoped I might find some freedom from it. I knew I had to find some way of getting into the sky; I had a felt sense that shivered through my body. And so, after the hike, I drove with Nick and Polly up to the Black Mountains Gliding Club, just a few miles from the farm, and bought a voucher to fly – one I knew I would use. The following week, I took that first flight.

*

The day after my first glider flight, I find myself climbing a steep hill that overlooks the airfield, and my mind is drawn back to the sky. Today, it is full of glory: an indescribable blue with pockets of fluffy cumulus clouds. Beneath them will be spiralling invisible thermals, reaching up through the sun's warmth – staircases in the sky. Walking on this hill makes me feel as though I am *under* the sky, and I realize that I felt at home during yesterday's flight, more comfortable in the unknown than in the known. What am I doing on the ground when I could be up there again? I rush back down the hill, skidding on stones, almost tripping, and head straight to the flying club. My timing is good; I put on an orange parachute, step into the glider and take my seat in the front. I am in the same sky-blue fleece and child's cloth sun-hat as the day before, and I am still in my mud-covered hiking boots; I'll be taking a clod of the earth up into the sky. Bo and I take off, tow up and release. I see the shadow of the glider crawling over the ground as we fly in circles over the hills and up to 3,000 feet.

Bo asks me if I want to fly and, this time, I say, 'Yes, OK,' a little tentatively. He talks me through it. My legs are stretched out in front of me and my feet meet two rudder pedals. I'm to place one foot on each. With my right hand, I take the stick, which is between my knees. Bo explains that the pedals control the rudder at the rear of the glider. Moved forward and back, the stick controls the elevator, also at the rear, which in turn moves the nose up or down, altering the speed. Moved from side to side, the stick controls the ailerons – long, thin flaps that stretch across the trailing edge of each wing. When one aileron is lifted, the opposite one dips. This makes the glider raise one wing and lower the other to 'bank' – to tip, in other words – and allow the glider to turn. Bo tells me to move my hands and feet in unison when I bank. Stick to the left, press left rudder pedal, and vice versa.

I must look out for any other aircraft at all times. I move my head in circles, scanning the sky above, below and around. I hold the stick in place to maintain speed, or 'attitude' as it's called.

'Look far, far away,' says Bo. 'Look to the horizon and maintain your attitude, the angle of the nose against the horizon.'

I'm amazed once again at the shapes of the ground from above. But this time I'm concentrating on the inside of the cockpit and I've less time to take in my surroundings.

Intending to bank to the right, I move the stick in that direction and notice the temptation to push hard with my right foot on the rudder pedal. The muscle memory in my right leg wants to push us forward with my foot, as I would by pressing down on the accelerator pedal of a car. So Bo decides to show me in visceral detail the profound difference between flying an unpowered aircraft and driving.

He tells me to come off all the controls. I take my feet off the rudder pedals and reluctantly let go of the stick. I clench my thighs. 'Relax,' says Bo, though I don't know how he can tell I'm tense from where he sits in the back. 'Clap your hands,' he says. I clap and then hear him clapping too. He stamps his feet and I stamp mine, muddy hiking boots clomping on the floor of the fuselage. Neither of us, nobody, is in control. We don't suddenly begin to fall out of the sky or veer off in an odd direction. We continue to fly forward at the same speed. The glider can fly itself. My job, Bo explains, isn't so much to control the glider as to correct its position in the sky.

A glider is always descending unless it finds air rising faster than it naturally glides downwards. Beside the rising air, a sort of downdraft occurs, where the air is being sucked under. This is the trick to soaring: finding air that's going up and then riding on it, surfing the sky. The skill is to manoeuvre inside the sky to find the lift – the energy that's already there in abundance, if you can only locate it. The challenge is being able to read the sky, to work out where the lift is and place the glider in it at the right speed to extract the most energy to stay aloft and soar like an eagle. This is what the buzzards I watch soaring over our valley are doing, I begin to realize: circling in rising air, which means they don't need to flap their wings to stay up.

'The whole sky is your engine,' says Bo.

I look out at the sky, full of bulbous cumulus clouds, and begin to see it differently. Perhaps it's not an empty space, a vaporous, gassy nothingness, but it takes an act of imagination to see it as a mighty force, a powerful engine.

'Go on,' says Bo, 'clap your hands. Clappety-clap.' We both clap and stamp our feet, and I feel as though we're applauding the very heavens.

I take the stick once again, rest my feet back on the rudder pedals and look ahead at the far horizon, where the hazy sky and hills blur together. I've the curious feeling of taking control and letting go at the same time.

Bo flies us in to land. According to the flight log, we were up for one hour and two minutes, but my sense of time was strange again; the flight seemed to go on for much longer.

On stepping out of the glider, I make a decision that clicks crisp and loud in my head. I want to learn to fly. I can sort of afford it. I have some savings and, for a few hundred pounds, I can join the club scheme, whereby I pay for the aerotows, but nothing for glider hire or instruction. I can fly only Monday to Friday, but that suits me; I am a self-employed writer not doing any writing. Bo is the weekday instructor, so most of my lessons will be with him. Everything in me calls out to do this. I have a deep sense that flying might become part of my recovery, a way for me to escape the grief of my illness and treatment. How to talk about the experience of cancer? I have been needing to find a language, a context, through which my suffering can speak, to make sense of what happened. Suddenly, in the sky, I have found a space for myself, a place to feel uplifted, so perhaps I will find my language in flying.

I fill in the forms and am given a flight logbook. Legally, I must keep a record of every flight I take, no matter how long or short.

As I walk out of the briefing room, later that afternoon, I have a new sense of direction all of a sudden – and it's up.

Chapter Two

Falling Upwards

My new-found desire to fly was shaped by a new relationship with the sky and its birdlife, which developed during
my cancer treatment. In the several weeks after the diagnosis, as I floated in the limbo between delivery of the
Bad News and the start of the dreaded Treatment, awaiting
phone calls that would announce further test results and
dates for hospital appointments, I left my rented home
in Oxford to return to the farm. It was July, and I spent a
lot of time lying on a sun-lounger cushion, on the grass
in the field behind the farmhouse, looking up at the sky.
I watched the birds and listened to the chattering of the
swallows as they swooped overhead, catching insects.

With this diagnosis, it was as though I was suddenly
thrown violently back into nature, reminded of my body,
and it was to nature that I looked for help. As I lay on
the grass, I was reminded of a Sylvia Plath poem, 'I Am
Vertical'. Plath writes, 'But I would rather be horizontal',
and goes on to say:

> It is more natural to me, lying down.
> Then the sky and I are in open conversation.

This is what it felt like to lie in the field, staring up into the blue. This catastrophic diagnosis was a call to begin a conversation with myself. I knew my outer public voice was already becoming silent, speechless. But, falling upwards, into the unchartered sky above me, a new voice began to whisper. 'I will hold you,' it said. 'I am afraid,' it said. 'You can collapse, fall apart, but you will remain.' I pictured the tattooed hands of an old sea dog with *hold* and *fast* written across his knuckles.

I desperately needed inner resources to cope with the ordeal that lay ahead, and the sky was a space into which I could fall upwards, where I could breathe. I pushed my mind as far up into the sky as possible and gathered its spaciousness down into me. Keep breathing, I told myself. One breath at a time.

*

My new focus upwards triggered a powerful dream that described my situation in perfect and subtle detail, as dreams can do sometimes. I've never been one to pore over my dreams, looking for significance; much of the time I can't remember them or they just seem to be surreal nonsense. But illness reached right into my subconscious, where dreams become vivid and meaningful. I was discovering that disease may manifest in the body, but it's a profoundly psychological, emotionally charged experience that shakes you right down to the bedrock. My imagination was starting to tell me stories about myself.

In this dream, it was night-time, and I was walking along the crowded seafront of a large city, the street busy with jostling people. The dark sky was lit by neon signs in garish colours – oranges, pinks, light blues. I was with friends and we were laughing. The seafront had a funfair atmosphere; games were being played somewhere and it was hot, sticky and tropical. Suddenly, an elongated creature, a sort of beast made of ectoplasm, grabbed me by my arm and yanked me into the night sky, rocketing me upwards like a firework. The creature pulled me into a dark-blue space between the stars, above, and the sparkling neon lights, below. We stopped there, suspended. The thing holding me up was energetic, mischievous and anarchic – a trickster; part Caliban, part Ariel. Together, we hung in the dark, moonless sky, and everything was still and silent. I was stuck, unhooked from the ground, my legs dangling in space. It was beautiful up there – cool, quiet and spacious – but I didn't know how to get back down to earth.

The dream had a raw, liquid, slippery truth about it. My imagination had conjured a little story full of images that expressed where I found myself and it stewed at the back of my mind while I waited for the treatment to begin. Meanwhile, I continued to look upward to the sky and birds for solace.

While I lay in the back field, on the cushion, watching the clouds grow and pass away, one of the five dogs we have on the farm would often trot past purposefully into the next field to pursue his private obsession. In a fever of excitement and frustration, he'd spend hours chasing swallows, running through the field with his head turned awkwardly skyward. He'd bark and howl at the birds as he ran, and they would tease him. They'd dip and weave, dive-bombing him, flitting just past his nose and behind his back to feast on the tiny white moths thrown up by his paws. Their agile flying easily outmanoeuvred his loud, clumsy leaps into the air.

Swallows return from their long migrations to Africa to the very barn in which they were born. Over the ten seasons of this dog's life, the sum total of his swallow catch was zero, and ten generations of swallows had learned this fruitful game. Later, when I faced the long, plastic tunnel of the M.R.I. scanner for the first of many times, this scene became a resource. Inside the dark tunnel, I began to feel constricted and enclosed, my mind started to fall inwards and then, suddenly, I saw the dog chasing swallows again. I watched him as he howled and leapt as black arrows dived and swept over him. Then I saw the blue sky above the dog and the swallows, and a sense of spaciousness opened up.

As my treatment progressed, and the swallows left for Africa, other birds became an important psychological resource, especially during the fiercely cold winter I spent enduring the deep horrors of chemotherapy.

The farm is surrounded by birds and perhaps that is because ours must be the only farm in Wales without a cat. We've had plenty in the past, but since the last one died, several years ago, we haven't replaced her. Dad refuses to have a cat on the farm any more because, each time one of them brought in a dead bird, especially a swallow, which is a holy creature to him, his heart would clench.

During that unusually cold winter of my treatment, we became snowed in on the farm for several weeks. Reduced to a wraithlike state, I was almost bedridden, so Dad put up a bird feeder outside my bedroom window. He made it in his workshop and then stood outside in the snow and blistering wind, in wellington boots and a blue hat, to set it up for me. I leaned on the windowsill from my bed, in my pyjamas, and gesticulated from behind the glass. This way a bit; no, back a bit; yes, there; right in my view; thumbs up. He knocked the bird feeder into the frozen ground with a sledgehammer and sprinkled birdseed on to it.

Dad replenished the birdfeeder almost daily, and over-wintering birds – such as nuthatches, jays, wrens, coal, blue and great tits, yellowhammers, robins, chaffinches and house sparrows – came to feed. Other birds that didn't come to the bird table were visible in the woods behind the house or flying past my window and sitting in the apple trees. Ravens cronked as they flew overhead, buzzards pew-pewed as they circled over the yard and owls hooted in the woods at night. We're on the migration route for redwings and fieldfares as they fly south. They stopped for a few days to feed on the 'Laxton's Superb' tree – a strange apple tree that keeps its fruit into the winter, long after all its leaves have gone.

One night, a fox, starving, scratched at the icy ground beneath the feeder for seeds that had fallen; we could clearly see her russet fur against the bright moonlit snow.

Propped up on pillows, bald and wearing two woolly hats, I watched these creatures pouring themselves into the task of surviving the brutal winter. I was determined to do the same, and I was grateful that we had no cat to undo the birds' labour of staying alive with a casual swipe of a paw.

On the farm, my family has to face death almost daily. And my dad knows how to use death well. Twenty years ago, he started replanting the orchard behind the farmhouse. Each lambing season, whenever a lamb died unexpectedly, as many do, he'd bury it in the orchard and plant a fruit tree on top of it. Some people put dry bone and blood compost on their gardens, so he figured that a dead lamb would be as good; he wastes nothing. One of the dogs would occasionally sniff out the lamb corpse and dig up the sapling to get to it, so we had to keep an eye on him for the first days after Dad had carried out one of his burial plantings. Now, many years later, as different fruits appear, I think of them as altered offal: plum-livers, apple-hearts, pear-kidneys. If you could take an X-ray of the orchard to capture the archaeology of the ground beneath the surface, an odd picture would reveal twisted tree roots fed through eye sockets, gripping young, toothless jawbones.

But my relationship with the dead on the farm became uneasy during my illness. I no longer felt a solid barrier between me and death: it felt too close, too possible. I noticed this when we found the fox. Shortly after my chemotherapy ended, when I was able to walk a little further again, we were collecting wood halfway down the farm and went to check the stream at the edge of the trees, near the top of a field. There, in a grassy opening, lay a fox. It was young and perfect, its thick shiny coat a flush of russet, with a big bushy tail. It looked as though it was asleep. It hadn't a scratch on it. I found the tranquil scene intensely disturbing, like a sign. I could barely look at it, but Dad was determined to have it stuffed.

He collected it, brought it back to the yard, wrapped it in a plastic sack and put it in the chest freezer in the stable. I thought of it, stiff and icy, lying on top of shoulders of our lamb and pork. Dad found a taxidermist in Ireland and sent the fox off in the post, and I thought of it, boxed up somewhere amid letters and parcels, slowly melting and beginning to smell. But the fox made it to the taxidermist and returned to us, months later, standing upright, one front paw raised, dead glass eyes and a dry scaly nose.

*

My internal sense of being suspended in the darkness, which had begun with the trickster dream, only grew as my treatment progressed, as all my hair fell out and I lost kilo after kilo, becoming so weak I could hardly climb the stairs. Inside, I felt exiled, stuck up on the edge of space, looking down longingly at the earth.

The Apollo moon missions have always fascinated me,

and, as the treatment continued, I became fixated on the Apollo 13 mission, in particular. It seemed to perfectly express my predicament. In 1970, three astronauts – James Lovell, Fred Haise and John Swigert – became stranded 200,000 miles from Earth, on their way to the moon, after an oxygen tank exploded. They were stuck in space for four days as NASA tried desperately to find a way to get them back. Images of the men trapped in their tiny ship would flash through my mind, making me wince in recognition. I was stranded, too, shot into space and in danger of never getting home, the hospital and Mum and Dad my 'ground control'.

At the peak of my Apollo 13 fixation, I discovered a pair of thick white socks in amongst the clean washing. They had *Apollo 13* and *Failure is not an option* printed on them. I didn't know where they had come from and they frightened me – a strange messenger, appearing from nowhere.

The most powerful part of the Apollo 13 story is how they finally returned. In order to get back, the astronauts first had to fly around the dark side of the moon, to get a slingshot effect from the moon's gravity to gain enough momentum to fly home to Earth. They had to go to the furthest, darkest, most remote place humans have ever been in order to find the energy necessary to return. In the worst moments of my treatment, when it felt almost impossible to endure it, a tiny part of me hoped that this darkness was the far side of my moon – a black place that contained a hidden energy source, if I could only work out how to use it to slingshot myself back to Earth.

Chapter Three

The Sky's Shadows

'You haven't seen a tree until you've seen its shadow
from the sky.'

Amelia Earhart

Driving the eight miles from the farm to the club most
mornings, a blur of bright colours rushes past me. It's May
and the banks have become long strips of multicoloured
wildflower meadow, of white lacy cow parsley, purple
bluebells, violet bush vetch, dark pink-throated red cam-
pion, white nodding mouse-ears, bright pink herb Robert,
golden buttercups and blue forget-me-nots, all highlighted
by a backdrop of dark-green ferns. There's one patch in
the bank that's thick with yellow cowslips, which flail back
and forth as I rush past them. I blow through this mass of
colour in a borrowed old farm vehicle, playing David
Bowie's 'Let's Dance' over and over again. I drive too fast
along the narrow, single-track lanes, the cow parsley and
ferns leaning over to obscure the view around bends
which already have little visibility.

The Black Mountains Gliding Club was formed in

1978, after a chance meeting between a local farmer and gliding enthusiast, called Derrick Eckley, and John Bally, a pilot and entrepreneur. Derrick and John worked tirelessly for several years to get planning permission for the club from the Brecon Beacons National Park. Derrick gave over a couple of high, flattish fields for the airfield, and removed some hedgerows and fences. Situated at the top of a valley, below the long ridge of the Black Mountains from Hay Bluff to Mynydd Llangorse, the airfield has spectacular views across Powys into Herefordshire and Shropshire, and over to the Beacons.

Soon after its opening, the club became renowned in Britain for having the longest national average flight time because of the ideal flying conditions here. Unpowered soaring flight happens best in hilly and mountainous regions because mountains shape the air around them and create invisible mountain ranges of moving air in the skies above. Pilots come from across the U.K. to fly, bringing de-rigged gliders flat-packed in long trailers that struggle through the narrow lanes to find the airfield, which is tucked away behind hedges, an old chapel and fields of sheep.

My flying lessons are between twenty minutes and two hours long, and most of them are with Bo. Born in Sweden, Bo spends six months of the year in Wales, teaching flying in the Black Mountains, and six months teaching in New Zealand. He hasn't experienced a winter for twelve years, which is a relief, he says, after Sweden.

As we speed at sixty knots along the ridge of the Black

Mountains, Bo explains the basics of free flight. There are essentially four kinds of lift we can use to soar, and all are the result of moving air, heated by the sun. Once you've been towed up, soaring is solar powered.

The first is ridge lift, where air meeting a hill or mountain moves up and over it to create an upward flow that can be ridden. That's what the buzzards that fly straight along the edge of the hill above the farmhouse are doing, I realize – riding the ridge lift. The mountains sculpt, mould, bully and funnel the air around and above them, much as a river bed, its rocks, curves and tree roots, works river water.

The second, thermal lift, is what creates cumulus, the lowest clouds – the kind that children like to draw, which look like fluffy cauliflower heads. These clouds are the result of warm, moist air rising from the ground. Unlike ridge lift, where you're chained to the hill over which the air moves, you can use thermals as stepping stones to travel across the sky, circling beneath one cloud, on the rising thermal of air that is forming it, to gain altitude and then travelling forward to the next cloud, and so on.

'The sky is powerful. Clouds must be respected,' says Bo.

I've often stood in the farmyard and looked through binoculars at swallows flying high above and wondered what they're doing up there, but I see now that insects get sucked up in these rising thermals, and the swallows follow them up to feast. My observations of the birds around the farm suddenly start to make more sense and my understanding of their relationship with the element they move in, the sky, begins to deepen.

The third type of lift is convergence lift, created where two air masses, gigantic or small, meet, and one will have to push upwards over the other. There are many different kinds of convergence lift.

Mountain wave, the fourth kind of lift, forms when air falls on the lee side of mountains and rebounds upwards, creating layers of invisible rising waves that reach high up into the sky.

So it's only possible to soar by having faith in something that's invisible: the air. You can feel the air you're surfing on, but you cannot see it. You can only see the air from its effects, and sometimes you can't see even those.

I begin to learn how to manoeuvre the glider in the sky by varying my speed – nose up to slow down, nose down to speed up – and banking and turning to stay in lift by moving the rudder and stick in unison. At first, I'm over-using the controls, jabbing at the stick, moving it too far this way and that, and pressing the rudder pedals too hard. Beginners often move the controls too much, Bo reassures me, like actors in a 1950s studio movie, pretending to drive a car.

Our glider is a K13, a steel cage in the shape of a canoe, covered with a canvas-like material called Ceconite. You could easily punch a ballpoint pen straight through it. The boundary between me and the sky outside is little more than the thickness of a jacket with a skeleton of steel supporting it, and I feel every bump and lift of this old sky boat.

Two giant eight-metre wood and fabric wings jut out from either side of the fuselage. Steel wires connect the ailerons, rudder and elevator with the rudder pedals and stick. Bo says it's 'a big old bus of a thing', but it's a good learning glider. The trainee pilot sits at the front, the instructor behind. There are dual controls and instruments, so either one of us can fly at any moment. In the front seat, my head is well above the body of the glider, sticking right up into the sky, and I feel it all around me.

The steel fuselage of a glider without its covering looks like the inside of a bird's bone: hollow, but cross-hatched with interior struts. Defying gravity is all about having strength without weight. The wings of the K13 are made of a central spruce spar and spruce 'ribs', so they're also mostly hollow. Spruce wood is often used in small aircraft because it's lightweight, flexible and strong. There's so little mechanics at work in a K13 that I can hardly bring myself to call it a machine, but the key is in the design, which is sophisticated. It's beautifully simple.

Because of its design, the K13 can act as a Faraday cage. A decade ago, Bo was struck by lightning while in the air. He was winch launching at another gliding club on a stormy day, teaching an architect to fly (a winch launch is when a glider is pulled up on a long cable by a winch on the ground, rather like a kite might be). At around 900 feet, Bo recalls a flash that seemed somehow to come from inside the cockpit. He felt a tingling sensation in the fingertips of his left hand, which was just touching the winch cable release knob. There was a faint, acrid smell of burning or of pure electricity. 'It's hard to describe,' he says. He realized immediately what had happened, released the glider from the winch and landed. Observers rushed over and said they saw the flash of lightning and heard a tremendous bang. Curiously, Bo doesn't recall any sound. The steel structure of the fuselage had acted as a Faraday cage, circulating the white-hot lightning around the two men and carrying it safely away from them, down the winch cable, into the ground.

*

Every morning at ten o'clock, Bo rings an old bell that hangs outside the clubhouse door to summon us all for the morning briefing, and we traipse into a small room beside the hangar to discuss the weather and schedule the flying lessons for the day ahead.

When I'm not flying, I help out at the club, as all club members are expected to do, towing gliders from the hangar to the launch point with a quad bike, helping to launch gliders by running the wing (holding and running with one wing tip as the glider moves off the launch point and picks up speed), and keeping the daily flight log.

Many people come to the club with vouchers for a single trip into the sky, and I often ask what motivated them to want to try it. Some say it's a birthday gift or some other celebration. One woman said her husband constantly has dreams about flying and this was the nearest thing she could think of to bring him closer to his dream-life.

The strangeness of being up in the air without the roar of an engine to act as a barrier between you releases conversation, even between strangers; it unlocks intimacy, vulnerability. I quickly notice how, with Bo behind me, our conversation is often unusual. And apparently it's not just me.

'All sorts of things come up,' says Bo. 'People say things.' Bo tells me that occasionally, during these one-off flights, someone will mention they're dying, usually of cancer. It makes sense to me that many sick people have an urge to get up into the sky, to look down on the earth they're preparing to depart.

When there's nothing to be done and I am waiting to fly, I sit on the edge of the airfield, watching gliders take off and land, and look up, trying to spot them soaring; they shrink and disappear, then reappear as dots that grow larger as they descend towards the airfield, trailing the signature high-pitched hissing sound as they come in to land. 'One can watch albatrosses for hours, like rough surf or fire,' wrote Peter Matthiessen, and this is also true of gliders.

The airfield is a helpfully in-between place to spend time, a beautiful grassy open space without much clutter. It isn't like a commercial airport, where people have onward destinations. This is a place where you can explore flight as something other than a means of transport, for its own sake. Our flight is unproductive and purely playful.

I had found it difficult to be around unfamiliar people during my cancer treatment, and I felt particularly vulnerable and transparent around strange men. If a man unknown to me came into the farmyard, I would often scurry and hide at the back of the kitchen or rush upstairs to peer out of the hall window until he went away. At the club, I am surrounded by unfamiliar men and I meet someone new most days. Every single one is kind, welcoming, helpful, gentle and generous with their flying stories, and I have eased into their company gratefully and made new friends. Nobody asks me too many questions about myself. We can just share a simple enthusiasm for flight.

The man with the most flying experience of anyone at the club, though perhaps not the most gliding, is John Coward, an eighty-two-year-old pilot. Aged nine, just before war broke out, his father took him to a flying circus, where he had his first flight in an aeroplane. From then on, he was hooked. As a child, he'd dream that he could 'run down the garden, flap my arms and take off.'

John has a long and varied flying career behind him, and has flown everything from Tiger Moths to Boeing 707s. He flew for several decades with the Fleet Air Arm of the Royal Navy, landing fighter planes at a hundred miles per hour on moving aircraft carriers. Later, he was a British Airways captain, and then he flew cargo planes all over the world in the 1980s. He flew live pigs from Vancouver to Johannesburg; live bulls from Khartoum to Yemen; and once newly minted banknotes from London to Bogotá, escorted by a troop of armed women who had flown in the day before and insisted on sitting in the cockpit with him. He even flew a Hunter jet to supersonic speeds (he told me that you don't hear the sonic boom, but a faint tremor of the shockwave comes through the rudder pedals and ripples along the wings to disappear over the tail).

He's a modest man, and quietly passionate about flying: 'I just like to be up in the air, and the feeling of being a part of the plane,' he says. John loves both powered and unpowered flight, but he says there is a difference: 'Power flying, it's just nice being up there looking out at the countryside, but you don't really feel you belong to anything.' He tells me, 'I never liked high-level jet flying on my own; it's a bit lonely up there at 40,000 feet. You feel cut off.' But he has had some fascinating experiences so high up, such as when he saw the Northern Lights over the Arctic Circle. 'The whole sky was lit up and they came right up to the cockpit,' he says. 'They were red, green and purple and so bright, it was like flying into the sun. You think you're going to fly into the lights, but they suddenly disappear at the last moment.'

He's also, on occasion, seen St Elmo's fire, a strange phenomenon of glowing static, often seen by sailors at sea during thunderstorms. 'It was like lightning inside the cockpit,' he says.

*

It is a still morning and, like surfers waiting for the waves to come up, club pilots pace the ground, longing for the weather to turn and become good for flying. People rig their gliders and carry out their pre-flight inspections. I wander into the clubhouse, where visiting pilots, club members and fellow flying students are drinking tea. The chatting runs and roams, moving back and forth with digestive biscuits and KitKats. Pilots tell stories of high flights and near misses, some knowingly exaggerated. In other stories, the risks and dangers are underplayed, quietly noted with careful understatement. Newspapers and magazines lie around unread, dirty teacups are scattered across the table. We are all waiting to fly. The jutting corner of Y Das, a giant chin of a hill, peers down into the clubhouse. We stand at the window and glare out at the sky every few moments. What's the cloud cover like? Is it raining on the ridge? How high is the cloud base? This is why unpowered flight is different: you can't just fire up your engine and go. Itching to get into the sky, we are already up there in our minds.

But the weather doesn't play ball, and the day turns out to be one for just hanging out at the club. And yet, as evening draws in, there is such contentment here. Two of the pilots stand side by side at the bottom of the airfield, looking up as they fly their remote-controlled model glider; someone is throwing a ball for a couple of sheepdogs; other figures are standing chatting at the edge of the airfield, whilst some go back to the tents and caravans they have pitched nearby, edging towards preparing dinner. Bo is cooking, singing along to 1940s Swedish folk music and making one of his perfectly soft omelettes. Later on, I join

Bo, Gary and some others at a local pub in the village below the airfield. Gary pulls up his T-shirt to show us his torso, which is tattooed from his chest down to his waist with the entire Welsh national anthem, written in Welsh. He doesn't speak Welsh and we all snort into our pint glasses.

*

The next day, the weather cooperates. I put on my parachute, buckle into the glider and feel on the edge of the sky. It's a hot June day, one month into my flying lessons; the sun beats down, magnified by the canopy into an orange haze that climbs into my eyes and clings around my neck. The sky is full of cumulus, moisture hitting the dew point and forming into unique shapes that have never been seen before. I'm learning to aerotow.

'Don't take your eyes off the towplane,' says Bo, as I try to fly in line behind it.

The ascent is bumpy; the glider rises and dips as we reach seventy knots. I push the stick too far to the right, which makes the glider swing out to the side of the towplane, creating a dangerous slack arch in the rope, which then tightens again with a jolt. Bo takes over and brings us back behind the plane. Aerotowing is tough, he explains; everyone finds it hard. He reassures me that, with repeated practice, it will eventually just click.

But the aerotow has real dangers lurking in it. If, when still close to the ground, a glider gets too high in relation to the towplane, the glider can pull the tail of the towplane up, forcing it to dive into the ground. Accidents are rare, but they do happen and I need to be aware of the importance of remaining level with or below the plane while on tow.

I release at 1,500 feet, above a series of ridges known collectively as the Dragon's Back (though its proper name is Y Grib), which descends in steps resembling a giant tail, reaching from Waun Fach down to the mound of Castell Dinas at its tip. The towplane falls away to the right; I slow to fifty knots, swallow, and look about for lift. Before we launched, the windsock on the airfield showed the wind blowing from the west directly on to the ridge, so there should be lift there. With Bo's help, I find it and rise on air currents pushing up over the hill, to double our height to 3,000 feet.

There's a peculiar physics and biology to banking and turning, which means that the landscape seems to move around us. The inner ear and brain don't register that it is our movement because the bank is cancelled out by centrifugal forces. If I was to take a cup of coffee up with me in the cockpit, it wouldn't spill during the bank and turn because the centrifugal force would keep it level in the cup (just as in any passenger jet). I've the curious sensation that the horizon is slipping past and that the hills are circling around us, as we stay still at the centre; they seem to rise up, kneel down and stretch out.

Cumulus clouds are forming across the sky and we explore the sliver of space between hilltop and cloud base, dipping and winding through a maze of thermals, being careful not to enter the clouds.

'If you fly into cloud in rising terrain, you will die,' says Bo emphatically. There are a number of known plane-crash sites in these hills, some from the Second World War, and most of those crashes occurred because planes collided with the hills in low cloud.

During these early flying lessons, Bo does the skilled work of keeping us in the lift so we can stay aloft and I can practise 'upper-air work'. We pass the controls back and forth between us, saying, each time, 'I have control.' We are not always peaceful. Sometimes, when the lift is difficult to find and we're losing altitude, Bo takes over and a stream of expletives cascades from the back of the glider: 'Oh, come on, you bitch!' he mutters at the sky, hoping I won't hear him.

'Are you swearing at Mother Nature?' I ask.

'Oh, no,' he says. 'Mother Nature is beyond all judgement and never has to give an account of herself. But an individual thermal, yes – she can be a bitch.'

Gliding is hunting, not for rabbits and voles on the ground, like a hawk, but for sunny spots that might produce a thermal, for ridge lift and rising air currents. It's about looking out, guessing what's going on, getting it wrong, trying again, swearing in frustration, yelling at the clouds and sinking ever closer towards the ground.

I begin to learn the basics of how to find and stay in the lift, which is done in part by looking for clues on the ground. I look at the windsock on the airfield before take-off to know the wind direction (though it might not be the same 3,000 feet above). Cloud shadows travel up rocky hillsides as outrageously shaped monsters, creeping along valley floors like intruders, and I look for the way in which they crawl across the land to see the wind direction at cloud base.

I look at the movement of ripples on water, on lakes or reservoirs, and at the direction I'm drifting against a chosen spot on the ground when holding the glider straight and level. Smoke or dust rising can also tell you the wind direction, and herds of cows and horses often stand with their bums into wind, so they too can offer signs.

Once I've established wind direction, I look for clues about where there might be thermal lift. Air above a ploughed field, Bo explains, will get warmer faster than air over grass; water rarely produces thermals; the air above bare rock or rooftops will heat up quickly in direct sunshine and can be a good source of rising air, as can tarmac and concrete.

Everything matters in trying to soar, and I must learn to pay attention to things on the tiniest and the largest of scales, from the black flecks of dead flies on the leading edge of my wings, which will affect their performance, to the cycle of the sun through the sky. We look constantly at where the sun is shining and on what, taking into account the time of day and time of year. An old disused quarry in the sunshine will produce lift in a way a river or lake will not. Afternoon sun shining on a south-west-facing ridge will produce much more lift than a north-facing ridge in the morning.

So, on one level, soaring without an engine is about stick and rudder, parachutes, glide ratio, ailerons, induced drag, audio vario and other instruments, but more profoundly it's about the way bare earth heats up compared to grassland at a particular time of day; it's about the way the wind blows, the colour of rock scree, the shape of streams and rivers, and the way a herd of animals stands against the weather.

There's no road in the sky. Each individual glider pilot finds a new pathless way through the air, a unique scribble. We locate a bit of ridge lift, here; fly out to a thermal, there; we wind and manoeuvre over the curving land. We never take the same route twice, so flight offers me a new perspective each time I fly.

As I learn to read the terrain for lift, I begin to notice more details in the ground below. When I am banking and the horizon slips past as we wheel around in a thermal, I hold the landscape in the corner of my eye. And in times when I'm not concentrating on flying, when Bo is working hard to keep us up, I look carefully at the land. All this intense looking unlocks new ways of seeing the ground.

Flying over the hills that surround our farm, I see a series of my many selves looking up. As I fly over them, they release particular memories, like exhalations. I glimpse my past on the hill with a strange clarity. There I am, as a child, exploring the mountain directly above the farm for the first time – a giant, wild world that seemed as big and limitless as the Sahara Desert to me. I see myself, a little bit older, running and sliding in wellingtons on the frozen dew ponds on the top of the hill in winter, laughter echoing across the ice, and the dogs chasing stones we threw on to the frozen pond, their legs going every which way until they quickly learned to dig in with their claws. I see myself racing Dad and the dogs along the flat path on the top of the hill, to the cairn at the crossroads of several paths, our rubber wellies making that mushy sound when we run in them, my chest heaving as I breathe in cold winter air.

Then I see myself as a grumpy teenager, lost and disorientated, on my own on the same hill, in fog, having proudly ignored an earlier warning from our neighbour, Ivor, who has lived in this valley and farmed since he was fourteen. 'Don't go on to the hill in fog because you will get lost,' he said, 'and don't sleep in the hay barn amongst the bales because you'll get "farmer's lung".' I ignored Ivor's advice on both counts. I remember wandering along familiar paths that had become different and strange in the mist, feeling certain that I was about to find the path that led back down the valley to the farm, but it never appeared. I eventually discovered that I was on an entirely different side of the hill.

At the remote top end of the farm, in the crook of the valley, I can just make out the stony colours of the ruined cottage that I claimed as a den for many years – a place to camp, hang out, make stinging-nettle tea with spring water and pretend to be a pioneer in a remote wilderness. I see myself camping there with my oldest friend, Bronte. She spotted an adder slithering between two stones next to our camp and I was upset that I didn't see it. We both burnt our calves on a metal plate kept too close to the campfire, which left us with matching scars. I often look for this scar when I'm in the bath, stretching my skin to search for some faint mark, but it has gone.

And there I am, in my late teens, one summer holiday, riding the unshod pony that came with the farm, used to herd the sheep from the hill in the years before quad bikes. I'm with a school friend, who's riding on another pony, and we're both wearing tightly wrapped T-shirts as hats to shield our sensitive redhead skin from the summer sun. We're squealing and galloping along the top of the hill, having just seen a man's naked arse sticking up out of the bracken.

Soaring over the hill opposite the farm, I see a family picnic with eighty-year-old Jim, my granny's cousin, one summer after I had left home and was visiting. Jim could barely walk, so Mum, Dad, my uncle and aunt manhandled him into a trailer, surrounded him with hay bales, cushions and blankets, and pulled the trailer to the top of the hill with the quad bike. We walked up behind the bike and watched as Jim bounced in the trailer, grinning, thrilled to be out of the nursing home and travelling to higher ground, for probably the last time.

I also see clearly the large field in which, as a child, I flew a big, bright-red stunt kite. On windy days, when the air rushed up the valley, we'd fly the kite here, away from the power lines. The Welsh cob ponies were sometimes in that field; they'd be spooked by the soaring red bird and would charge back and forth along the hedge line, their wild, unkempt manes and tails flying. I didn't mean to scare them, but secretly I loved watching them gallop and hearing the thud of their hooves, a racing pulse coming out of the ground.

Standing, holding one string in each hand, letting the kite out as far as possible, it was as though my mind travelled out of my fingertips, all the way up the string to the weaving kite, soaring in the air. I'd imagine looking back down at my upturned grinning face. The tugging feeling of the string pulling my arms felt like an urge to follow and rise skyward.

And so the sky has become a new, groundless place from which I can look at where I've come from. I am gaining a fresh perspective on these memories, and it feels wonderful.

Beyond my own memories, other dimensions of this landscape appear differently from 1,000 feet up and more. At different altitudes, different timescales of the past appear. It's as though the air is stratified.

Between 1,000 and 2,000 feet, a history of farming is written into the crazy-paving patchwork of fields and farms below: a big field with one corner lopped off and joined at an awkward angle to another; three tiny fields jostle for space next to one four times their size – this is the parcelling up of land between sons and brothers. Each farmhouse is nestled into the hill, away from the harshest prevailing winds, the windows often turned towards the east to catch the dawn sun and get the farm families up and moving. It's clearer from the air how villages and towns huddle around rivers. I've an aerial perspective of how the landscape works: it's less a series of isolated farms to me, now, and more an interconnected network.

And it seems smaller, too. I now see more clearly its delicacy and the way each part is connected to another. The logic of human design, anchored in the land and climate, is visible. I look below at the shapes we have made for ourselves to live in – houses, gardens, schools, chapels and churches. They look fragile from up here, even though many of them are hundreds of years old and built from thick, unmovable stone walls. They seem more like barnacles clinging to a ship.

Lots of ruins, many hidden or inaccessible from the ground, stand out from up here, too, and occasionally, when low, I can see the strange forms of trees that have grown inside their abandoned chimney stacks.

We navigate by two such ruins that sit a mile or so to each side of the airfield. To the north-west, the ruined landmark is an abandoned mental hospital, a group of stone buildings halfway up the valley. Out on its own amid open fields, it's a solitary site, abandoned to the hill; the landscape seems slowly to be reclaiming it. The building looks like a stark and obvious metaphor for the minds it once housed, as though the very walls took in the broken-ness of its patients and are now exorcizing it in their own crumbling.

On returning to the airfield, more often than not, Bo will begin the preparatory circuit by saying, 'Head towards the hospital,' or, 'Over to the hospital.' It's strange to begin my descent back to earth each time by passing over the stone shell of an abandoned psychiatric unit; the ruin reminds me of my own psychological fragility, and looking down on it makes me see how far I've already come.

To the south-east of the airfield is Castell Bwlch y Dinas, meaning 'fortress at the pass'. From above, it's a series of circular ditches rising up the mound at the base of the Dragon's Back. Shadows seen from the air pick out a ground indented; hedges encircle the mound, clearly marking its circumference. Built at 1,476 feet, on the pass between the Black Mountains and the lowlands, Castell Dinas, as it's known, is the highest castle in both Wales and England. It's my 2,000-year-old waymarker; if I can't find lift, when I see Castell Dinas, I know it's time to head back to the airfield.

Sometimes, my view from the sky allows me to see even further back into this landscape's history. There are ancient and subtle man-made marks on the land from the Neolithic strata of time that are only visible from the air at particular times of the day, if the light is right. Neolithic long cairns or burial barrows are scattered across the land and they appear when the sun is low, in the afternoon, casting long shadows that just pick out the shapes of earth-works. Ripples, dents and ditches caught in a certain light stand out as we fly low over the ground, and, though I'm uncertain what exactly is there, the shapes are obviously man-made. A shadow passes briefly across a bit of rough ground and then disappears again, like a half-remembered moment flashing across the mind.

At higher altitudes, almost all human marks disappear and a vastly different layer of time surfaces – a geological one. The twisting paths of the gouging glaciers that moved through this landscape are visible and I can see where they ground downslope, creating U-shaped valleys and bringing giant frozen boulders to carve and scrape out the bowls at the base of the hills.

From 3,000 feet upwards, the hills become a long, continuous sweep, and it's impossible to say where one hill ends and another begins: Mynydd Llangorse, Pen Tir, Mynydd Troed, Twympa, Y Das, Waun Fach, Pen Allt-mawr. From the ground, I can name individual hills and I know their unique shapes well, but from above, what I see is the wider pattern of geological repetition across the whole body of hills. The Black Mountains are like plump seals, much softer and more rounded than the Beacons, which, in contrast, have hard rock escarpments jutting up out of them, like the hips of an aged bony animal.

*

The first time I fly the landing, a dozen lessons in, I don't know I'm doing it. Bo doesn't tell me I'm alone on the controls. Once we've reached the ground, rolled forward along the airfield and come to a stop, he lets me know it was all me, and laughs when, elated, I make him promise he is telling the truth.

The most dangerous part of gliding is the landing. It's the ground that will hurt you, not the sky. Stalling and falling out of the sky close to the ground is the danger, and the exceptionally small size of our airfield in the Black Mountains means you must come in steep and watch your speed. If you fly too fast, you might overshoot, and if you're too slow, you might stall. You only have one chance to get it right because you can't power up and go around again.

It's summer, and every lesson, now, I fly the landing. We edge around the airfield, passing over the ruined hospital to line up in the correct position to land into the wind. Coming in to land, the earth rushes towards me, I pull gently back on the stick to hold off the moment of meeting the ground, and we skim over the tips of the grass blades before descending the last few centimetres and feeling the wooden skid beneath gently bump down on to the earth. We roll forward along the airfield. From the back, I hear the stuck record of Bo's voice repeating, 'Wings level, wings level, wings level.' I grip the stick and feel the wings wobbling from one side to another. I make small adjustments to bring them back to level, as ordered. The tips of the wings must not hit the ground while the glider is moving at speed. If they do, you can 'ground loop', where the wing tip catches the ground and pulls the glider suddenly and jarringly around. As we roll along the grass, after I've flown us into a smooth landing on a particularly blustery day, I hear Bo mutter the word, 'Fearless.'

*

That evening, as I am driving away from the club, back to the farm, I realize that, every time I fly, I have the feeling of being swallowed whole by the sky and spat out on landing. I come back different, remade, but it's a shock to be on the ground again. I think about what Bo said, that I was fearless, and perhaps I am, to the point of recklessness. I am happiest up there, flying where there is width, depth, space to explore, and suddenly the ground has become just a jumping-off point, a means of getting to altitude. I may have learned how to land, but, now I've begun to explore the sky, I'm not sure I want to come all the way back.

Chapter Four

The Wilderness Above Our Heads

It's a sunny day in late June and most of the pilots who have come to fly are already in the air. Waiting for my lesson, I wander into the hangar as several swallows leap from a perch on the metal wall and fly all over the hot interior. They've recently fledged from a nest tucked behind an iron girder. The metal walls creek, crack, click, snap and tick as they expand in the heat. I stand in the middle of the hot hangar and watch the birds fly all around the space, over white, outstretched sixteen-metre wings, dipping, weaving and turning in flight, so fast and agile it's hard to see them clearly. The gliders are covered in bird droppings, especially the Slingsby T21, an old 1940s open-canopied aircraft that looks like a classic sports car with wings. It's stowed directly beneath the nest. It's impossible to keep the swallows from nesting in the hangar, so every-one is forced to clean the droppings from the wings of their aircraft each morning. The giant sliding hangar doors are ajar, but the fledglings aren't yet ready to leave. This large metal barn full of aircraft has become a swallow nursery.

There are birds all around our gliding club, and we

watch them with that eternal human jealousy that birds arouse in us. Adult swallows swoop overhead, catching flies; curlews nest at the end of the airfield and make their distinctive high-pitched warbling whistle as they fly away, down the valley. I look up and see a red kite and a crow fighting in the air. The kite circles slowly, banking this way and that as the crow, half its size, squawks and dives at it. They look almost entangled for a moment, then the kite slowly moves away, flapping its big wings, and the crow flies off in the opposite direction.

While I wait my turn to fly, Keith Richards, the club's maintenance engineer (we've also got a club member called Neil Young), offers to take me up in his Europa, a two-seater powered aeroplane. It's a still day, and we rise quickly to 3,000 feet, the propeller spinning invisibly ahead of us. We fly down the wide valley at the edge of the main body of the Black Mountains and back over the Brecon Beacons. I stare down into dark, stony moss-coloured valleys as we fly straight and fast over the hills. The engine is loud and it's hard to speak, even though we are seated side by side.

After thirty minutes or so, as we are heading back towards the airfield, a crackly voice comes on the radio. I can't make out what's being said, but Keith registers something. He flies on past the airfield and descends. I look down and see one white wing tip sticking up out of a field of tall dark-green grass. I stop breathing; it looks to me like a glider has crashed into the field. Keith says,

'There he is,' and I see a man walking along the edge of the field towards a gate. It's Bo. He's not crashed, but he has landed out. I breathe again and we fly straight back to the airfield and land as several people are preparing to retrieve Bo and the glider. A few of us bundle into Keith's car, someone else tows a glider trailer and we set off.

We arrive at the edge of a field along a dirt track, half a mile off a narrow country lane, to meet a furious farmer, understandably distressed by a glider landing in his field of valuable crops. His face is red and he stomps around, shouting as Bo apologizes and explains that any cost will be covered by the club. The oat crop has been flattened in an area slightly larger than the glider, where the wings have moved over the grass as it landed.

A group of six guys disassembles the glider, removing the wings, canopy, elevator and rudder, and we carry each part down a half-metre-wide path through the crops, trying to tread as little of the grass underfoot as possible. This will be my gliding lesson for today.

Back at the airfield, sitting in the clubhouse, Bo explains that, on his way home, he had got into some surprisingly strong sinking air and he had had to make a quick decision and find somewhere to land; he knew he wasn't going to make it back to the club. He chose the best option: a field level enough and large enough to land in, with no power lines, livestock, barns or streams. Bo had been taking a man for his first glider flight. His wife had bought him two flights for his birthday. Bo had calmly told him at the very last moment that he was going to land in this field, and to hold tight. The man never returned for his second flight.

I am amazed at how unfazed and calm Bo is. Landing out is a part of all unpowered flight, he explains. If you fly out across the country, even experienced pilots will often find themselves without lift and be forced to find somewhere to land. That's why he tells me to 'always have a landable area in mind. Always have a plan B. You must always be looking for somewhere to land if you need it.'

And now I have time to think about the flight with Keith in his little power plane. It was curious to cover so much ground and sky in so little time, and with such ease. The depth of the experience of trying to stay up without an engine, and soar, was gone. To me, it felt like crossing a patch of ocean in a powerboat when you usually sail; the skill, effort and relationship with the elements was all lost. The power flight felt flat, linear and metallic compared to gliding. Soaring in thermals, we circle and spiral, rise and descend, making shapes that are liquid and malleable, always more fascinating to me than straight lines.

The relationship with the undulating terrain and sky was totally different too. It was odd to spend time in the air *avoiding* turbulence. I have been getting used to gliding inside the sky, following the contours of the landscape and seeking out unstable air to find lift. To me, instability means staying up. So, oddly, the alarming site of Bo's glider landed in a field hasn't put me off. Always looking for somewhere to land while soaring will simply sharpen my awareness and observation of the landscape below.

After that day, I start to notice clear, flat fields without power lines cutting through them everywhere.

*

The following day, I'm back up in the sky without an engine. Flying along the west-facing range of the Black Mountains with Bo, who is totally unruffled by his land out the day before, we see the herd of feral ponies that live on the hill, running beneath us. As we creep out of the ridge lift and tip into a thermal that seems to run up my legs and into my spine, I glance up and spot a buzzard just above us. The bird doesn't appear to see us. It soars over my head, circling round and round in ovoid shapes, banking just as we do. I crane my neck upwards and see the soft white and brown speckled underside of its feathered body and its elegant outstretched wings. I am trying to take in everything, holding my breath and opening my eyes wide. I want to hold on to this moment. The tips of its primary wing feathers are splayed-open fingers, pointing to the sky. I watch as its dark-brown wings make small adjustments this way and that, twisting up a bit, down a bit, responding to every tiny shift in air current. The bird is so supple in the air, it moves almost like water. I can see that its scaly black claws are closed together and tucked back. So often, I stand in the farmyard, peering up at buzzards circling over the valley. Then, they're remote black crosses, far away in the distant sky. Now, I'm right up close to one, exploring its world with it.

Suddenly, the buzzard glances down and sees us;

alarmed, it panics, seems to wobble in the air, draws in its wings and dives down steeply, off to one side, away from us. A surge of excitement rushes through me and I feel the thrill of a trespasser.

Higher, now, and out over the valley, away from the hills, black flecks dart and spark across my view, only just visible, whizzing up and down, back and forth, up here at 3,000 feet. They're swifts or swallows, or both, that have ridden the afternoon's strong thermals to gorge on insects sucked up by the columns of rising air.

Flying on over towards Y Das and the Dragon's Back, I spot another bird, but this time we are above and looking down on it. It's a red kite, soaring slowly into the wind, close to the steep edge of the mountainside. It's almost still above the ground as the air rushes over its wings. The muscular curve of its shoulders is visible and, unlike the buzzard's rounded tail, the kite's russet forked tail flicks sensitively, responding to the shifting air currents with a liquid flexibility. The red kite's body is still, but its head moves constantly back and forth, up and down, remaining acutely aware of what's going on all around and below, looking for every tiny rustle in the undergrowth with its sharp eyes. I'm envious of its flying skill and the ease with which it moves about in the air. To look *down* on a soaring bird is astonishing; I never dreamed it was possible to see a bird up close in this way, soaring along with it, using the very same flying principles and energy in the sky.

But I'm particularly excited to be flying close to a red kite because of their history. The sky was empty of red kites when I was a child. I never saw them on the farm or over the hills above. In fact, the red kite has only recently been brought back from the brink of extinction in the UK. Persecuted from the sixteenth-century Vermin Acts onwards, they were extinct in England and Scotland by the turn of the twentieth century. Only a few pairs remained by the 1960s, living in the old oak forests of Mid Wales. Concerted efforts, from the 1960s on, to feed and protect the red kites, and more recent reintroduction programmes in Scotland, England and Ireland, have meant that they're now living wild in all areas of the British Isles once again. The first sighting of a red kite in London for over a hundred years was reported in 2006.

Now, we have several that circle over the farm, along with the buzzards. They must be nesting nearby. When Dad cuts the grass for hay with the tractor, red kites join the buzzards to follow him, looking for mice, voles and frogs torn from the safe cover of long grass. But, where the buzzard will sit and watch the tractor from a fence post or tree, Dad told me, the kite will fly over the tractor, following it. He knows it's there when its shadow washes across his face.

When I see that russet fork-tailed bird slowly circling, mewing in its piping, whistling call, I see hope as well as magnificence. 'Hope is the thing with feathers,' wrote Emily Dickinson. The red kite has come back and recovered. It shows that things don't always just go in one direction: stories can turn around. Losses can be undone.

Soaring birds are helpful in our flying, as well as a

tremendous treat to observe. 'Always look for hawks,' says Bo. 'They will guide you. They know where the lift is, better than anybody.' I'm pleased to hear him use the word 'anybody', because, in learning to fly without an engine, I feel like I've entered the realm of the birds. After my illness, it feels only right that I should look to them for guidance.

*

As well as looking for soaring hawks and other birds that catch a ride on rising thermals, I look to the clouds for lift, especially to the cumulus clouds, which mark the thermal tops.

A cumulus cloud floats past to my right. It's slow moving, or so it seems, but it's hard to tell up here. I'm flying at about sixty knots, but I don't feel the speed. I watch the cloud, wispy at its edges, white mist against the cerulean sky. I pass by it, or it recedes behind me – I can't tell which. Neither can I tell whether it's growing and forming, or slowly melting away. I bank and circle on the edge of the cloud; the ragged edges of it touch over my right wing; I dip beneath and look up at it, wraithlike above me in its milky paleness.

Once I'm past this cloud, things speed up again. We're back to sixty knots. I need to slow down to stay in the lift of the thermal that's feeding this cumulus cloud, now above me; I'm trying to remain beneath the cloud in the rising air. I pull back gently on the stick, a millimetre or two, reducing my air speed to fifty knots, and begin to circle underneath the cloud.

The air moans. Since I've started learning to fly a glider, many people have asked me if flying without an engine is as quiet as it looks from the ground. No. It's noisy as hell. In the old K13, the air howls loudly all around and whistles into the cockpit through hair-thin gaps where the canopy meets the fuselage. The audio vario, the instrument that tells you if you're ascending or descending by the tone and speed of its incessant beeping, begins to beep faster and at a higher pitch as I rise in the thermal lift. It should be an annoying noise, but now I associate it, Pavlovian, with the good news of rising air and gaining lift. *Beep . . . . beep . . . . beep . . . beep . . . beep . . beep . . beep . beep . beep beep*, it goes, as the needle on my altimeter winds around clockwise, showing that I'm gaining height.

It's hot inside the cramped cockpit, so I open the vent to my left and feel a rush of cold air against my cheek. The stick is clammy in my hand. I turn my head to look out to the left for any other aircraft, but all I see is an ocean of cumulus clouds, slow-motion waves rolling above the undulating landscape, their shadows down on the ground exploring, fingering curiously the curves of the hills, before being swallowed down rabbit and foxholes, and cracks in rocks.

Bo tells me to look out across the whole sky for the larger emerging patterns of clouds, for places where 'cloud streets' are forming along ridges or down wind lanes – long strips of cumulus clouds that we can soar beneath.

A fat, dark-bottomed cumulus looks likely to be a tall cloud because it's blocking more of the sunlight, and therefore it might have a strong thermal beneath, feeding it. But it might also mean that the thermal is running out of steam. So it's important to look for the wispy beginnings of newly forming cumulus clouds, where a rising thermal has just met the dew point and is condensing into water vapour.

Despite all of these clues in the clouds, much of the sky is still invisible, so I must try to imagine what's happening, to build a mental picture of what's going on around me in order to guess where I might find the energy to stay up.

The gases that make up the sky are continually recycled and partially created by the very life forms the air sustains. Oxygen, carbon dioxide and nitrogen, the gases that make up the majority of the sky, are in an infinite feedback loop between the air and the living and dying organisms on earth that it protects. The sky is a virtuous circle, the earth's airborne circulation system, mirroring the rivers and seas below. The air warms, rises, cools, falls, blows and spins across the whole planet, and circulates water, as well as dust particles, pollen, fungi spores, bacteria, insects and birds, all carried across vast stretches of the planet.

Though the sky may seem enormous from where we stand, it's also terrifyingly thin, in terms of the scale of the planet. The life-giving troposphere, the lower of five levels of atmosphere identified by scientists before we reach outer space, is on average a mere seven miles thick. From sea level, heading vertically upwards, you could walk to the very edge of the life-sustaining sky in a few hours. Passenger jets ascend through the troposphere to fly at cruising altitudes at the bottom of the stratosphere, at around 30,000 feet. No clouds form up there and only the most powerful storm clouds grow tall enough to poke through. Flying just a few thousand feet up with a good 20,000 feet of troposphere left above me, the sky seems enormous, infinite and oceanic in size. But, on a planetary scale, it's a thin layer of cellophane wrapped around a watermelon. Seven miles and below is all we've got to live in, and that is the business end of the sky, as far as free flight is concerned. This is where the weather happens.

It's hard to appreciate the powerful energy in the sky from the ground, except perhaps on a particularly windy day. On a still day, the sky can seem remote, empty and unimportant, a background hum to the real matter of life on the ground. But that is an illusion. A single cumulus cloud is a floating lake, and weighs as much. It is water stripped of gravity. The energy in the latent heat of an average-sized cumulus cloud is the equivalent of approximately 300 tons of TNT and a giant cumulonimbus storm cloud contains the latent heat energy of a nuclear warhead. A 'cu', as pilots call a cumulus cloud, is a collection of opposites: it's heavy and yet it looks light; it's full of powerful energy, but appears flimsy. 'Vaporous', 'hot air', 'wind': all are words related to clouds, which also mean 'insubstantial' or 'empty'. But these words are misused back on the ground because, as gliders know, the thermal that creates a cu is pure energy and substance.

In time-lapse film footage of the sky, it's possible to see how it broils and roils, rises and rolls over itself, growing clouds that pass away like great, giant waves. Moisture cools and mushrooms, seemingly out of blue nothing, and then tumbles over other clouds and disappears. Winds travel at different speeds and in different directions at various altitudes and, in time-lapse footage, we can see the different air masses clashing and merging, falling apart and regrouping. Our human timescale doesn't allow us to see the dynamic energy at work in the sky.

Bo is teaching me to look at clouds and imagine what might happen next, to fast-forward in my imagination and guess where the best lift is. I'm banking in a steep turn, my right wing tip pointing to the hills below, which are dark green, now that it's summer and the fern is fully out. I'm observing the sky and then imagining how it's working where it's invisible. Bo encourages me to 'guess and go there, feel your way into it. Nose around the sky.' I don't see a thermal, but I can feel it as soon as I enter it, and I try to focus, to feel whether I'm inside it or falling out of it. I understand, now, that when Bo goes quiet, he's concentrating not just on looking out at the sky and imagining it, but also on the subtle feel of it. There's something of the swell of the sea in this sensation.

Many pilots have described gliding to me as three-dimensional sailing (in the U.S., gliders are called 'sail-planes') and, as I start reading some classic aviation books, I find that many power-pilot authors experience flying as navigating a floating ocean. Antoine de Saint-Exupéry's *Night Flight* is filled with descriptions of planes as boats, and he writes a gripping account of flying through a thunderstorm, which he describes as like a ship sailing through a stormy sea; he compares a calm sky to an aquarium, and, flying over South America, he looks down on the land as a seabed. In *West with the Night*, Beryl Markham describes the trusty two-seater aeroplane she flies across the plains of Africa as 'a bright fish under the surface of a great sea.'

It's the same for me. Focusing on the sky, the earth recedes and becomes a seabed; an area of woodland is a coral reef, the ruins, shipwrecks, and the swallows, swifts, pigeons and blackbirds flying beneath me are fish exploring it all. The buzzards and red kites are slow-moving sharks, swimming above the reefs.

And, like so much of the sea, the sky is a wilderness. We cannot truly own or permanently inhabit the sky, farm or harvest it; in fact, it's barely accessible, but it's always there, just above our heads, moving, shifting, bringing the weather and constant change.

The sky certainly stirs my imagination, spurs it on and gets it going, and flying inside it, thinking about what's going on out there that I can't see, I can't help conjuring some of its many ancient and stubbornly persistent mythologies.

Watching sunrays burst through clouds one afternoon,

casting golden fingers of light on to the emerald-green ground below is almost too much, almost ridiculous. I've entered some strange Christian celestial moment. Flying beneath a big, bulbous cloud, it's easy to assume that, coming out around the other side of it, I'll see a cherub bobbing about on its top. Flashes of witches on broomsticks, archangels, wrathful Greek gods and mythological flying horses pass through my brain as I circle and weave through the sky. From 3,000 feet up, rainbows appear regularly and I see them from above as the sun glances through the water droplets in clouds. It's like flying inside a child's drawing, and feels both clichéd and fantastically new.

The inaccessible sky has always been a space into which we project our imaginings of things that feel real, but which we can't see. I've heard the word 'sky' is from an Old Norse word, 'skuggwa', which means 'mirror' or 'shadow'. Our way of naming the sky has persistently been connected to the reflections and projections of the human imagination. Look up into the sky and see for yourself. Like the old ink-blotch Rorschach tests, we see in cloud shapes what's already in our heads: faces, bloated bodies, dancers in slow motion, animals running, crawling and swimming across the sky.

And yet, now that I'm learning how to stay up and soar in the actual sky, it's becoming the very opposite of ethereal. The closest I've come to the feeling of soaring before is swimming underwater; it shares the sensation of being held up, and the sense of a three-dimensional, morphing immersion. What had seemed remote and empty is now intimate and full. The air becomes as thick as fast-running water; I can feel its strength through the movement of the glider and, on some days, it feels chewy, elastic – a thing with texture and substance.

My right lung, scarred from radiotherapy, feels the pinch of cooler air, and I picture this slight stabbing sharpness as the icy blue of the sky reaching down into me. On each inhalation, the air grasps me from the inside, and, on each exhalation, it lets me go. The idea of the sky as the realm of an unearthly heavenly kingdom and disembodied spirits seems wrong now. The sky has become earthy, physical, both inside me and all around me; I am bound in its body.

*

The more time I spend in the air observing, in ever greater detail, what is happening in the sky and on the ground, the more I start to notice the sun's movement across the sky. And, with this renewed awareness, there also burns into me a new sense of time and place. I feel the season in the strength of the sun's warmth, the time of day in the angle it hits me, and my direction of travel in which side of my face it's shining on. In one moment of heat on my skin, the sun becomes a felt calendar, clock and compass.

Many pilots, I notice, are like this; they just know what compass direction they are heading in all the time, in the air and on the ground. It has become instinctive.

Driving through the narrow lanes, I glance in my rear-view mirror and look up at the sky above and behind the car. There is a giant cumulus cloud growing and the sun is shining through the back of it. It is summer, mid-morning, must be eleven-ish. I know I am heading roughly south-east.

Later that day, I am helping Mum and Dad with the shearing, out in the field by the barn. I collect up huge fleeces, waxy yellow with lanolin, and lay them out on a trestle table; I fold in the legs and tail of each one, rolling it up into a woolly ball to shove into the giant sacks of fleeces to send off to the wool board. The dogs pant in the shade as they watch the sheep being undressed. My hands are oily and the sharp animal-sweat smell of raw wool sticks in my nose. Lanny, the local farmer who comes to shear our flock each year, is bent over a ewe, halfway through shearing her, when he looks up and asks the time. Neither Dad nor I wear a watch, but we both immediately turn our heads to the sky; we know the pattern of the sun as it moves daily around our valley.

'Twelve fifty,' says Dad.

'Twelve thirty,' I say.

We later look at a clock and we were not far wrong. Approximate time is perfectly adequate here; we've no trains to catch.

This renewed sense of place and time is slowly relocating me in the natural world, and although I am sailing up in the air whenever I can, I am also beginning to feel more grounded in natural processes. It is a relief, because a painful sense of being unnatural grew in me after my cancer diagnosis. Cancer made me feel excluded from nature because I became ill so young, and, after diagnosis, my body felt alien – a mutant, rejected from the natural order of things. Now, though broken and scarred, I am re-establishing a place for myself, I am finding my way back into the natural world through time. Flying without an engine, human and clock time seem to disappear as a new kind of time surfaces, one that is natural and multi-layered and changes at different speeds and at different altitudes. Like the movements and route of an unpowered flight, time seems to have become rounded, curving, circular, spiralling, connected both to the shapes on the ground and to the rhythms of the day as the sun arcs across the sky.

Flying time is both stretched and shrunk. On landing, a two-hour flight seems to have passed in an instant and yet each individual moment of that flight was huge and full.

'A glider pilot makes about four decisions every second,' Bo tells me, and perhaps it's this concentrated decision-making that expands time for us.

When I mention this time-warping to other pilots, many acknowledge that their sense of time changes in the air too.

'Time passes more quickly,' says Mike Codd, a fellow club pilot, 'especially flying cross-country, when you're so busy reading the sky and making decisions.'

Time seems to disappear altogether for Bo. When teaching flying, he wears a watch to time the flights. 'Sometimes I don't know if one minute or ten minutes have passed, so I have to look at my watch to keep track,' he says. 'When you are flying, an hour can go by so quickly . . . You don't realize it . . . Your focus removes your sense of time passing.'

The Greeks identified two kinds of time: chronos and kairos. Chronos is man-made time, clocked and calendared. But kairos is something different, something altogether more unruly and unpredictable – a shape-shifting, wild time. When flying, a variety of timescales within kairos seem to open up to me, but, in truth, before I started to learn to fly, I was already remote from chronos. Illness totally blew apart my previous sense of time, and, during my treatment, I discovered dimensions of time that I'd never felt before. Moments waiting silently for the results of a scan seemed like a painful forever, and each long, slow day crawling through the side effects of chemotherapy was a giant frozen clock face.

But I could take advantage of this slowing down, too. I could sit silently by the fire in the kitchen, while Mum and Dad cooked, watching the dog sleeping, his breathing body lit by the flames; I watched birds at the feeders outside the kitchen window, and from my bedroom, with great attention, noticing every jerky movement as they hopped about with nuts in their beaks. Such ordinary things were transformed by my focused attention into moments of wonder, inside which I found enormous resil-ience, and therefore slow, painful time became a resource to help me get through the treatment. In the days leading up to a chemotherapy session, I'd savour every moment as a way of slowing the time down and holding off the appointment for as long as possible.

I now know that time can warp and bend, speed up, circle and deepen, depending on what you do inside it. Part of my way of psychologically healing myself after cancer, knowing that I've to face the horror of ongoing tests for the rest of whatever length of life I have, is to rearrange my relationship with time. Flying offers me the means to do this, enabling me to confirm this sense of the subjectivity of time, and, crucially, strengthening my ability to expand it. I am learning to inhabit and stretch time, to dive into it rather than skim over its meniscus surface.

*

I circle beneath a cloud in a thermal and Bo tells me to slow my speed to stay in the lift. I pull back a millimetre on the stick and slow to forty-five knots; the air quietens; I look down at the green Dragon's Back with the brown slash of the sheep track, worn larger by hikers weaving up its spine. The hill seems to rotate beneath me. I feel at the very centre of this moment, full and fat with life.

The past and the future recede to tiny dots. I imagine a cross-section of a second from up here. So much happens: my heart beats, as does Bo's, as do hearts across the ground below, of people, birds, sheep, horses, foxes and other wild animals hidden in the undergrowth, and night creatures sleeping underground and in tree hollows. I breathe out, thousands of other creatures breathe in, a swallow flies past, a tree branch waves, wind full of dust, pollen and bacteria brushes my face, something decays a little bit, something grows a little bit. Every single second is wide and vast, and we've got 86,400 of them a day. Each second is a little infinity of its own.

Chapter Five

Navigation by Scarlight

'For nothing can be sole or whole
That has not been rent.'

W. B. Yeats

'This is why I do gliding myself, to get actually into
the air itself and get a further sense of depth and space
into yourself, as it were, into your own body.'

Peter Lanyon, painter and glider pilot (1918–1964)

There's no blue in the sky. It's a windy summer day, full of
big rain-shower clouds. The sun is blotted out as they pass
overhead, but the air is unstable, dynamic, and this means
that the ridge will work well, if thermals are hard to come
by. We set off into this glowering sky, I do the aerotow
well and we soar relatively low in ridge lift merged with
small thermals. A shower falls and raindrops run up the
canopy as we push into the wind, blurring the view of the
hills below. Sudden turbulent thermals shove and bump
my back, rippling up my vertebrae.

I'm learning to do something that feels counter-intuitive: move towards and into the turbulence. Flying into the edge of a thermal, one wing is pushed up by the rising air. Instinctively, I bank away from it, wanting to move out of the lumpy air that shoves and jolts. But, in order to find the energy in that turbulence, I must do the opposite and turn towards it, move into it and try to put the glider at the very centre of the unstable air to ride up on it.

My hand and foot coordination on the stick and rudder is still off and unbalanced, too jerky and hurried because I'm trying to over-control the glider.

'You're a subtle person,' says Bo, 'so be subtle in your movements on the controls. Move the stick just a milli-metre, wait for the ailerons to take effect, respond rather than react.'

I try to relax my thighs, where tension seems to accu-mulate. I'm not nervous, but I am frustrated with myself and want to get it right.

'A smaller input sooner is better than a bigger input half a second later,' Bo explains. 'Don't move the controls unless you have to.'

As we head back to the airfield in the rain, Bo tells me to stop looking down at my instruments so much. 'Your head should not be in the cockpit, but out there in the sky,' he says, adding, 'We'll cover them up.'

'What do you mean?' I ask, thinking I've misheard him.

'The instruments,' he says. 'You don't need them at the moment, while you're learning, so we'll cover them up.'

Intrigued by this idea, I spend an afternoon at the club, a few days later, making a rudimentary instrument-panel cover. I find an old magazine lying around the clubhouse, tear out a few pages and place them in sections over the instrument panel of the second K13, which is in the hangar today. The pages show adverts for upmarket gentlemen's clothing: corduroy trousers, woollen jumpers and leather shoes. I cut the paper around the T-shaped edges of the panel to make a template, and then find an old cardboard box and flatten it. I lay the template over the largest section of cardboard. It just fits. I cut around the template and paint the board black on both sides with a tube of cheap acrylic paint from home. I leave the panel in the sun to dry.

A day or two later, I take my black cardboard panel to the launch point, along with a roll of electrical tape. It is a hot July day and the grass on the airfield is shimmering in the afternoon heat, turning the trees in the distance, down in the valley, into a wobble of rippling greenery. I put on a parachute, climb into the front of the glider and fasten the panel over all the instruments, one piece of tape attached at each corner. Where there had been a series of round dials, an airspeed indicator, altimeter, compass and variometer, there is now nothing but a flat black blank. I must rely on my ears, eyes and the rest of my body to work out what's happening. I feel excitement tinged with anxiety, naked without any instruments to go over on my preflight checklist.

As Bo and I take off, I realize that the high-pitched

beeping audio variometer is also missing. It must have stopped working. There is really nothing mechanical to tell me what is happening in flight.

I manage the aerotow well and release at a good height above the hills (though I'm not certain what height exactly). My concentration is absolute. The sky is cushioned with cumulus clouds. Insects lifted up inside the thermals splatter in yellow streaks across the canopy of the glider.

Bo has his instruments in the back uncovered. He tells me to guess our speed and, to my surprise, I guess it quite accurately from the angle of the nose against the horizon and the sound of the air rushing over the wings: fifty-five knots. I slow down to forty-five, and the noise drops.

I soon begin to really feel the full push on entering a thermal and the pull downwards on leaving it, and I'm finding that, thrown back to rely on only my senses, I can trust my body to know where I am in the sky.

The left wing is pushed up, so I know that's where the lift is. I bank, turning the glider into the invisible and unstable rising air. The wing tip angles further and the glider ascends; I feel the rise in my stomach as a slight tensing. My spine is lifted very slightly too.

I eyeball the peaks and mountain edges. It takes practice and experience to know instinctively the length of the wing, and therefore how close it is safe to fly to the hills. I'm not nearly there yet, so I keep my distance.

'The danger is that new pilots are sometimes tempted to pull up on the stick and slow down, precisely the opposite of what you should do when flying close to the ridge,'

Bo explains. If you slow, there's a danger of stalling, and stalling close to the hill is not a good idea. You must do quite the opposite: speed up and drop the nose, when flying close to a hill, to make sure you don't go anywhere near the stall. Flying without an engine sometimes requires you to do the opposite of your untutored instinct.

This is pure flying! I feel completely inside the sky, eyes up, looking out properly for the first time. I'm untied from the rope of numbers and the false sense of security gained from measuring things. Let go of the instruments, my body is in the glider, but my mind is released. I land feeling blown open and off balance by this flight, shredded by the wind, but happy. The only thing to do is to pursue this unravelling.

For the next several flights, I use my instrument cover, reattaching it with fresh tape each time I strap myself tightly into the K13. Nobody else wants to use it, and as they help me launch, there are always some fellow club members who look askance as I cover up the instruments.

Flying without the instrument panel means I must turn my attention inward to feel what my body is registering, right down into the depths of my lightly churning guts. I can never feel the details of the movement of the air very well to start with; it's like a dull sensation, muffled, as though felt through a pillow. But, as I attune, I'm able to concentrate more fully on the feeling of lift and sink, and they gradually get 'louder'. The feelings are always clear on entering a strong thermal, but in weak lift or sink, the sensations are subtle and difficult to feel.

On occasion, Bo will say, 'There it is – can you feel it? Turn now, turn, turn!' yelling from the back, and when I don't notice anything, I feel deaf and blind and insensitive – a blunt instrument. At those times, my legs still push too hard on the rudder pedals, and I slap and pinch my thighs in frustration, trying to sting them into doing less. But I'm getting better at it. 'You have to feel the air in order to progress,' says Bo.

I have bought an inflatable, pocketed cushion – called an 'AirHawk', appropriately enough – because my bum goes numb after forty minutes or so in the air. The multiple pockets of air in the cushion move and rise a little as we bump through some lift or sink or rotor turbulence, so it's my butt, as well as my inner ear, guts and spine, that provides information about how to stay up. Learning to fly unpowered is a visceral experience and my whole body is slowly becoming a flying instrument.

Illness taught me to distrust my body. I felt perfectly well when I found the first lump, but after the diagnosis I realized that, in truth, I really had no idea what was going on inside me, beneath the skin. The whole treatment was a kind of out-of-body experience, from which I haven't yet fully returned. During the treatment, I had to focus on the psychological dimension of coping with it. My job was to build what I think of as a little bird's nest in my imagination, in which to house my mind while my body fell apart. Learning to really feel the new sensations of lift and sink, I'm undoing some of the work of illness and re-entering my body, re-possessing it and learning to trust its signals.

Learning to fly is a process with trust at its core – trust in the engineering of the glider, trust in Bo, who passes trust forward to me from the back seat in bite-size pieces, teaching me to put trust in myself. With the instruments on display in front, it's tempting to take this trust and quickly throw it forward on to the panel, like a hot coal, never pausing to feel what my senses have to say. But, right now, I'm learning to rely on my own judgement.

*

By the end of August, flying without instruments has become standard practice for me. The whole landscape has taken on a yellow hue from the cut fields where farmers have made hay, the round, black plastic-wrapped bales gathered at the edges, and the tops of the hills are dry and pale. Our hay is all made – small, square, sweet-smelling bales – and stacked in the shed.

I fly into the edge of a cumulus cloud and, remembering Bo's warnings, bank to get out of it. I'm only inside its wispy strangeness for a few seconds, but as I come out the other side of it, I'm shocked to find that, where I thought the ground was horizontally below me, it's in fact tipped beneath at a steep angle. I've discovered the one place where I cannot trust my body to fly.

'I have control,' says Bo, as he brings us well away from the hill and the cloud. 'Inside a cloud,' he explains, 'most people will not know what's up or down within thirty seconds of entering it.' With no visual reference or horizon, a pilot quickly becomes disorientated and the brain and body start to tell lies. The liquid in the inner ear provides an idea of what is up and down, but once the pilot is in a steep bank, blinded by cloud and with no visual clues, what feels like up is probably an angle of bank of thirty degrees or more.

Warning me about cloud flying later, back at the club, John Coward says, 'Your inner ear will give you all the wrong sensations and tell you you're doing things you're not.' This is especially the case if you turn in a cloud for any length of time. 'You can easily get to a stage where you have no idea which way up you are.' And once your brain has decided what's happening, he explains, it won't let go, seeking confirmation of what it assumes, which is most likely to be wrong.

Neither powered nor unpowered pilots can fly in cloud unless they have trained to fly using only their instruments, including an artificial horizon. Crucially, the pilot must learn to distrust what the body and brain says is up or down. I glance through the books scattered about at the club, including *Human Factors for Pilots*, in which I read up further on the problems of orientation for pilots flying in and out of cloud. There is a chapter on 'Spatial Disorientation', which explains that 'there are a number of ways in which the pilot can suffer from illusions of orientation,' including interpreting a sloping cloud bank as a level horizon, or a pilot might even 'misidentify ground lights (perhaps a flotilla of fishing boats in a featureless sea) as stars.' Our brains and bodies have not yet evolved to fly, and we easily misread and misinterpret our experience in the three dimensions of the air, our inner ear throwing our visual clues out of whack with our sense of balance.

I soon come to realize that, in powered aviation, the pilot essentially learns progressively to distrust the physical and sensory information received in the air. 'The only solution to all forms of spatial disorientating,' the chapter concludes, 'is for the pilot to trust the most reliable form of information available to him; this will almost invariably be his instruments rather than his own sensations.'

Unpowered flight is quite the opposite: the glider pilot must learn to distinguish between embodied information that's useful and trustworthy, and that which is an illusion. Yet again, I'm reminded of how different free flight is to powered flight. The useful sensations in the flying body will help the free-flight pilot stay airborne.

*

My family and friends might see my flying as escapism, as a distraction from the pain of my illness and separation, and from my fear of the future, but the truth is otherwise. Learning to fly, I'm getting more intimate with this pain. Up in the air, I'm released from the claustrophobia of that tightly crowded little island below, where there doesn't seem to be space enough to feel. Soaring at altitude might look from the ground like a form of escape, but in truth it's my way of piercing the surface of my pain and going underneath, into it. Strangely, I'm experiencing altitude as depth.

Attuning to my body's feelings of flying takes me

inward in ways I've been resisting. It's impossible to really concentrate on the felt sense of flying without being confronted by emotions I've been unable to face thus far. They are feelings trapped inside my body in the same places that register the sensations of flight.

I have to really concentrate in order to learn to fly, and this absolute concentration becomes the still eye of the storm, around which an emotional whirlwind begins to spiral during flying lessons. The hard rock of grief inside my chest is still there, heavy and solid. It is still overwhelming. I don't know what my place in this world looks like any more, but, if I can feel, then perhaps this is something, some way of re-entering.

Learning to fly without an engine is providing me with a much needed meta-narrative for my recovery: I need a story beyond the confines of the N.H.S., doctors' letters, pink leaflets on hormones and survival statistics, nutritional advice and metal sheets of pills. I need more than that for it all to have been worthwhile. Being left with a scar, a repeat prescription, a signed doctor's note and an annual check-up simply isn't enough. I need a useful story to inhabit, and this is precisely what learning to fly is providing.

I circle around and around, like a red kite, gazing ahead, and feel an inward expansion. Intense pain wells up from my chest and, softened by the sea of the sky, passes through me and is released out into the blue, where it dissipates. Perhaps this is what freedom really is: room to feel the full stretch of your emotions, and then to let them go. Where the ground has a tendency to close me down, to fence off my emotions, the space up here gives my pain room to breathe. The sky is big enough to hold any amount of grief.

With the help of the sky and the clouds, I have started to explore my pain in small doses.

Once the wave of pain has been fully felt, extended as far as it can go, the edge where it finishes becomes clear. And, having found the edge of the pain, there's now room for other feelings to begin. As ferocious emotion pulses through me and out into the sky, it's often followed by a hot flash, a burning silver bolt of intense joy. Pain, it turns out, moves through the same inner networks as rapture. When one moves, so can the other; if one is blocked, so is the other. This is the victory of brokenness. 'What is to give light,' wrote Viktor Frankl, 'must endure burning.'

I surrender to the pain that surfaces when I'm at altitude in the same way I surrendered to my illness and its treatment. After the diagnosis, many kind and supportive people told me I was in a 'battle' with cancer, and would advise me about the skills needed to 'fight' the disease. It was a language of violence and conquest. I was encouraged to 'know my enemy'. I took quite the opposite approach: surrender, gentleness and vulnerability. In not fighting, I found a quiet attentiveness to the present moment and an intense intimacy with the world that revealed a raw toughness at my core, which gave me enormous strength to endure.

Now, instead of lying on the ground and throwing my

mind up into the blue to look for help, I am immersed in the sky, feeling its movements right down inside my inner ear and up my spine.

As this embodied sense of flying deepens, the very boundaries of my self are beginning to stretch. The subtlety of the movements needed to keep the glider soaring is starting to settle into my body: the tiny corrections with the toes on the rudder pedals, the small movements to right and left, forward and back with the stick. As I relax more into the glider, and as my confidence on the controls improves, my body and the flying canoe begin to blur together. Where my feet finish and the rudder pedals begin becomes less defined; my spine seems to reach right down and back into the wings that jut out behind me. The strong steel cables that attach the controls seem to extend out of my fingers and toes, are metal tendons that stretch into the elevator and rudder at my rear. The glider starts to feel like a kind of flying exoskeleton.

I talk to other pilots about this and almost all agree that, as the student's flying improves, when the learning moves into muscle memory and flying starts to become instinctive, the places where the body ends and the aircraft begins become indistinct. And this goes right back to the beginning of flight. Wilbur Wright, the older of the two brothers, suggested that 'By long practice the management of a flying machine should become as instinctive as the balancing movements a man unconsciously employs with every step in walking.' With this in mind, on warm summer days, I sometimes fly barefoot, throwing my

shoes into the hedge at the edge of the airfield before climbing into the cockpit. With my bare feet working the rudder pedals, I feel even more connected to the aircraft.

*

I've been flying for five months now, getting to know the sky and the hills from above. But there is one part of the landscape that troubles me. I bank steeply, circling in a thermal with my wings almost vertical. The horizon tips and, at one point in the circle, my lower wing tip points down towards a dark patch on the hill that I haven't allowed myself to look at since I started to fly. Each time, I turn my gaze upwards as soon as the burn scar appears, and look past it to Waun Fach, the highest point in the Black Mountains. I usually engage fully with the landscape, so it's been strange to find a part of the land that I cannot bear to look at. I have my reasons.

Flying over the Black Mountains is to fly over a giant body of hills that sometimes, on days when my imagination is particularly porous, seems like an extension of my own body. I look down and see a tangled arrangement of thighs, hips, arms, backs. As I bank and turn, the hills rise up, spin around, lie down, bend, bow and arch. The landscape looks alive and breathing.

Inspired by my enthusiasm for gliding, Dad takes a flight with Bo; it has been twenty years since he had those few first flying lessons and took the photo of the farm from the air. After his flight, he says that, from above, the hills remind him of Henry Moore sculptures. Moore's

sculptures blend the British landscape with the human form, one wrapped inside the other. It's as if the hills mirror bodies that mirror hills.

This is why I can't look at the scar on the hill as I fly over it: it reminds me too much of my own.

I say nothing to anyone about this, I can't find the words to talk about my preoccupation with the scar on the hill, but during conversations with pilots at the club, I slowly discover that the scar is a landmark that people navigate by, both in the air and on the ground. It is used as a point of location by locals who hike, cycle or ride these hills on horseback, a way of orientating themselves in the landscape. The patch is not on the map and has no name, but it has a vivid presence in the minds of all who live close by. The burn scar is visible from many directions, above and below the hills, from the sky, from the road that winds just below the hill and from several miles away, towards the village of Glasbury. On landing and being asked where he flew, a pilot might reply, 'To the burnt patch and then along to Hay Bluff,' or, 'Oh, not far – in and out of the bowl of Y Das and over to the burn.'

I haven't been able to look out of the glider at the scar on the hill, in the same way I haven't been able to look in the mirror at my own. When I see the patch out of the corner of my eye, as I drive along the winding lane towards the gliding club, and refuse to acknowledge it, I have been refusing my own.

But now I have an instinct that I need to look down at the scar on the hill when I fly over it; I know that, if I can just face it, I will find something I need there. During the next few flights, weaving along the ridge, I force myself to purposely look at the scar. My stomach is knotted as I peer down on it, but I hold my gaze steady, and, over a series of flights, my curiosity begins to grow and it gradually becomes a little easier to look at the dark scar.

The burn is about an acre in size and covers the top of a hill called Pen Trumau. 'Pen' means 'high' in Welsh; when I read the name of this hill on a map, I just read *High Trauma*. It is a patch of peat that burnt for weeks during an unusually hot summer in the 1970s. Very little grows there now, even forty-odd years later, and the wind and rain rub away at the peat, further eroding the side of Pen Trumau. Time does not appear to be healing it.

One day, flying over the scar on the hill and glancing down at it, I notice a distinctive white line crossing the black peat from one side of the patch to the other. I wonder what on earth it could be. Back at the club, I discover that the line is made of sheep's wool. Exactly a month before I began to learn to fly, the 'Woollen Line' project was launched to do something about the bare patch. A local artist and conservationist decided to try something new in an attempt to encourage regrowth over the scar and prevent further erosion. She had the innovative idea of pegging rolls of sheep's wool into the scar in rows, to hold the peat in place, and then sewing seeds into the wool. The Gurkhas, the highly skilled Nepalese regiments of the British army, train locally out of Brecon, twenty miles from Pen Trumau, and a group of them helped to carry the heavy fleeces on the steep five-mile hike up to the scar, from the nearest road. Then volunteers staked the rolls of white wool into the black peat with wooden pegs. A bright line of wool, thick with lanolin oil, ran along the scar in an undulating shape.

The burn goes so deep into the ground that, even if the wool does help plants to regrow and stops the peat from washing away, the scar will likely be visible for a long time. The black patch cannot be unburnt. But perhaps just being able to hold my gaze on the scar on the hill, not turning away from it, could be a kind of healing – one that doesn't require the scar to disappear.

I need to get closer to the scar, so I decide to visit Pen Trumau on foot. I set off one August morning from the airfield. As I get closer, I am almost afraid to approach it, as though it might suck me in and swallow me whole. But when I reach it, I tentatively sit down on the patch, catching my breath. It is a hot day, blue sky, a cool breeze at my back, which is sticky with sweat from the hike up. A glider sails overhead, passing in front of the sun for a second and casting its shadow over me. Its wings create a high-pitched whistle. The skylarks sing.

I lie back on the dark ground and stare up into the blue.

The peat is warm to the touch, and the wool has rotted into it. I stand up and wander all over the scar, the peat soft and yielding underfoot, squashing like a chewing mouth sucking at my hiking boots. Cracks run along the peat where it is dry, opening up fissures within the already scarred ground. Nothing is growing here yet.

I let the scar on the hill guide my thoughts. Nobody knows how the fire started, but if it was simply the summer heat, then this scar appeared through natural processes. The more I look at it, the more the scar on the hill and my own scar start to seem like openings for painful truths to enter. Illness is a part of nature, as are hill fires. Wandering around on the bare peat ground in the midday heat, I try to accept the inherent fragility of the natural world, which includes myself. And, with this on my mind, I hike back down to the club and head for home, knowing I need to think more about the scar on the hill.

*

Since I started flying, I have been writing. I write down the basics of each flight in my pale-green pilot's logbook, filling in the titled columns with nothing more than the date, glider type and registration, the launch airfield and time in the air. But there is one line for 'Details of Flight'. At first, I stuck to it; I was just keeping this log for legal reasons, after all. I wrote perfunctory details, such as 'Ridge lift' or 'Good thermals' or 'Hot sun', but recently, putting pen to paper for the first time in over two years, other than to sign medical consent forms, I have begun to run on to the line below, noting more and more details about each flight, squeezing them into a few short lines with ever tinier handwriting.

I find an old unused A4 sketchbook in my room at the farm. I take it to the club and, after a particularly good one-and-a-half-hour flight, I open it, grab a Biro and, sitting on the bench in the clubhouse, I begin to scribble. I describe the flight in as much detail as possible: what I saw, learned, all the sensations, physical and psychological. Suddenly, language cracks open again; it is as though the sky has moved through me on to the page. I write scrawled notes that are private love letters to the wind. The urge to write is exhilarating; I thought it had died during my illness.

Now, when I land, I'm itching to write while I can still feel the lift – flying and writing have become entwined. I finish one notebook and start another. They are the origins of this book. The words come by themselves, from somewhere I guess we'd call the subconscious. Influenced by the ancient seam of human thought that associates the sky with the imagination, weaving and circling in the sky begins to feel like sailing through the realm of the subconscious itself. The conventional spatial model has the conscious mind layered over the top of a subconscious that lies beneath. Exploring the sky, this begins to seem like a wrong-headed model that we've dragged into fact through continual use. I've the idea that the subconscious encircles the conscious mind, as the blue atmosphere encircles the rocky planet. This image feels satisfying and right. It's a spherical, planetary model of the mind which nicely does away with notions of above and below. It's all rounded.

Pilot and writer William Langewiesche says of the relationship between flying and writing, 'when we do not understand the weather, we may pretend that we do. Flying as much as writing teaches the need for such fictions, for discerning patterns in a disorderly world.' To write, for me, is a kind of flying, and flying is a kind of writing into the sky, a surfacing of heart and head, a learning again, a reworking of internal connections between all the parts I might call myself. In both learning to fly and beginning to write again, I'm finding some way to navigate the chaos.

Chapter Six

The Fascination of Wings

'My mind is not a vessel to be filled but a tinderbox
to be set alight.'

Plutarch

FLIGHT FOUR

Wild surrender, up and into the sky. Above the fields,
above the hills, sailing like Egyptian gods in this oceanic
sky, over a prehistoric earth. Wild heart, open and hurt
facing into the wind; I let my pain rise up to melt into
the shape-shifting cumulus clouds. They are never still,
never caught or trapped. I let the wind carry me, push
me, tidal, wide-eyed, falling and rising. I am the glider. I
am the horizon. I am the wind that lifts me, I just didn't
know it. There I was, all along, reaching up, falling
down, getting it wrong, pulled by the gravity that keeps
us suspended between blue and green. Move, fly, swing
around, dive, spiral up, turn back, upside down in an
ancient arc – the sky is beneath me and the earth hangs
above. Up here, I am letting the wind ride through me,
making a hole for the sun to shine into. I can play. I can

trust in the intimacy of the elements, the thermals and ridge lift, the invisible and the unfathomable nature of the wind. I can trust in my own nature and his and everybody else's. Yes. Say yes. Why not?

He whistles behind me, a tune I half recognise.

from Notebook four

I focus on nothing but flying, think about nothing else, talk about nothing else, read about nothing else. My once-brief notes on my flights are now long passages of euphoria. Nothing on the ground interests me very much. I am irritable in landed conversation, I don't like visiting towns, I don't listen to the news or read a newspaper. I have cut myself off from the outside world and, in doing so, feel more connected to the place where I am.

Fellow club members say they've seen it all before. 'It's a marriage-breaker,' says Mike, and I think, Yes, but my life is already broken, and I feel more alive in this brokenness than ever.

I climb into bed each night in a state of impatient excitement about the following day. It is a feeling I haven't had since childhood, and the intensity of my learning seeps into everything. Now, I fly to sleep, conjuring the skies through which I've flown during the day, my flying lesson replaying from take-off: the soft jolt as I release from the towplane, gravity pulling during a steep banking turn, and the bump of turbulence that I feel up my back on entering a thermal.

It is as though I fall to sleep on the wing, roosting in the sky.

I am having flying dreams again. No longer stuck up in the night sky with a trickster, or trapped in space; in these new dreams I fly free, willing myself into the air by sheer power of thought. I fly over railway tracks and peculiar glasshouses, people staring up at me from the ground, quizzically. In one dream, I fly with my arms outstretched and come in to land just like a glider, controlling my speed and getting ready to run.

Most days, when I wake up, I jump out of bed and put on the clothes I wore the day before, left in a pile on the floor, where I stepped out of them. I run soap and water over my hands and face before heading straight out without eating.

Driving the eight miles to the club too fast, peering up at the sky over the steering wheel, my whole body twitches with anticipation. I've no thought other than to get airborne. Each landing is merely a pause before I can get up there again.

Sometimes, when I land, a rush of strong emotion pulses through me and I have to run off the excess energy. Children are allowed to run because they're bursting with energy, but adults can only run if they're jogging on a fitness regime, or in a hurry. I am too embarrassed to say I just need to run, so I charge back and forth a few times across the airfield, pretending to be fetching something for someone in a rush to launch.

Lifting my knees, pushing with the balls of my feet,

pumping my arms, feeling my heart beating faster in my chest, memories of being too weak to climb the stairs after chemotherapy flash through my mind. Feeling well and fit enough to run is a glorious miracle, a moment of intense pleasure still to be had on the ground.

I am reconnecting with childhood in other ways too, and I begin to realize that flying reminds me of many exuberant sensations from my youth. The feeling of lifting up on take-off has an echo of being on a swing, when it reaches its furthest point and pauses for a second before it lets go and reverses to drop in the opposite direction.

On the farm, Dad made a rope and branch swing, attached to a big old oak at the top of a steep field. We'd pull the branch seat far back, until it almost touched the ground, put one leg either side of the knot, cling to the rope and push out to swing forward and watch the ground fall away. Everyone wanted to try it, including my diminutive eighty-seven-year-old grandmother. Shortly after she had her turn, the branch on which the rope was tied broke off in the middle of the night.

Flying also reminds me of my somewhat alarming childhood habit of leaping from rooftops. Dad had a single-storey workshop next to the back garden in our first home. It was sunk down into the ground a half metre or so and one wall had a ledge part-way up, so that, if I stood on it, age eight, I could just about haul myself on to the flat roof. I remember well the urge to jump off. I wanted to fling myself out into the air. And each time I'd plan to do it when Mum and Dad weren't looking.

Standing upright and surveying the garden below, I'd raise my arms and bend my knees, like a diver facing the edge of a high diving board, pause for a moment, take a deep breath and then push off with both feet as hard as I could. I'd jump out above the garden, arms and legs flailing, my body a star shape, trying to keep aloft for as long as possible. I would jump without screaming or whooping, silently flinging myself into space. My body can still recall the feeling of having let go of the rooftop, of charging out into the air, of the exhilarating surge that combined a little bit of fear with the knowledge that I was doing something naughty. A rushing white noise filled my ears as I anticipated meeting the ground. I'd remind myself to bend my knees and roll on to my side like a parachutist just descended from the clouds. Then I'd hit the grass with a thump.

I must have spent a single second in the air – two, at the most – but this time is expansive and thick in my memory, the feeling stored in my body, coiled up somewhere like a spring.

Between flying lessons, I start to read up on the history of free flight. I want to understand the origins of this strange and fascinating activity, and I discover that I'm not the first person to have an urge to leap from high places. Many of history's tower jumpers and steeple leapers, as they're known, leapt in an attempt to fly.

In 1862, George Faux, a farmworker from Essex, climbed on to the roof of the local pub, wearing nothing but a pair of underpants. Faux had watched the birds and believed it was the way the front edge of their wings cleaved through the air that enabled them to fly. This brought him to the conclusion that he could fly by beating his bare arms. He rapidly hit the ground.

Much earlier, in 1507, an Italian named John Damian had tried to impress King James IV of Scotland by leaping from the walls of Stirling Castle bedecked in homemade feathered wings; he said he would reach Paris faster than the King's ambassador, who had just set off overland to France. Damian broke his thighbone on crash landing, and later explained that his failure was a result of using chicken feathers instead of eagle feathers. In 1610, a Russian named Vliskov jumped from a high building in Moscow, clad in wings made from linen and eagle feathers. He too plunged to the ground, but survived.

My favourite British steeple leaper is Eilmer of Malmesbury, an eleventh-century Benedictine monk who made himself wings and leapt from the abbey tower in front of spectators at Malmesbury, in Wiltshire. He was fascinated by the story of Daedalus and thought it based in fact, so he sought to replicate the Athenian engineer's feat by building his own wings. Eilmer is recorded by the chronicler William of Malmesbury as performing a substantial glide from the tower, travelling 'more than a furlong', nearly seven hundred feet, his monk's habit flapping. He landed badly as a result of 'the violence of the wind' and his 'consciousness of his own rashness'. He broke both his legs and limped thereafter. 'He used to relate as the cause of his failure,' wrote William of

Malmesbury, 'that he had forgotten to provide himself a tail.'

Eilmer became known as the flying monk, and there's a stained-glass window in Malmesbury Abbey that depicts him holding a model flying machine, looking off wistfully into the distance.

There's a childlike exuberance in Eilmer's story that I relate to and which I have come to associate with the urge to fly with the birds. Learning to fly feels like an extension and development of that part of me that loved homemade swings and leaping from the roof of Dad's workshop, which I now see is perhaps a universal human urge, one that fuelled those early tower leapers. Free flight allows me to express a simple, direct euphoria at being alive that had slowly withered and eroded as I entered the self-consciousness of adolescence. The horrors of my cancer gave me a way to let that self-consciousness fall away and be discarded. During the long, arduous treatment, I stepped out of my memories of an awkward adolescence as out of an old dress, and, instead of moving forward, I went backwards – or was it sideways? – and rediscovered something of my prepubescent exuberant girlhood.

Riffling through Mum's drawer of photographs, I found, along with the picture Dad took of the farm from a glider, a photograph of me, aged about eight, on holiday in Spain, wearing a swimming costume, flat chested, grinning with gappy teeth. I now feel stripped back to this earlier self. I recall being fearless and unselfconscious at that age, throwing myself at new adventures. It's as if this strange experience has twisted time back on itself and I've been offered a backward glance at childhood, allowed momentarily to return there to draw strength from it.

This feeling has been made acute by the nature of the farm. The farmhouse has changed considerably since I left home. Solid stone walls have disappeared, replaced by doors or windows; a stone spiral staircase has been transformed into a cupboard with shelves; an old oak screen has appeared from beneath plasterboard; a stone bread-oven has emerged from behind a cast-iron wood-burner; the white house has turned stone-coloured, and the steps up to the front door have been moved around to the side. But, outside the shape-shifting farmhouse, much has stayed exactly the same. The same rusty horseshoe hangs above the stable door; the same hole is in the dry stone wall, next to the gate into the garden.

And the organic world beyond the farm seems to have changed hardly at all. The walnut tree at the bottom of the yard has grown only a few centimetres in every direction in the years since I left. The course of the brook falling down the bottom of the valley has moved to the left a bit here, to the right a bit there. My childhood is intact, here. The past isn't another country at all.

The small size of the passage of time since my childhood is most visible in the ash tree at the very bottom of the farm, on the edge of the known world, as it was then. The trunk is hollow, but the tree is still alive. Friends and I would climb up the metre-and-a-half-high trunk to the opening into its hollow centre, and then descend into the blackness, terrified and amazed. Our tense, excited voices echoed in the musty chamber where rings of time had once been, but had rotted out, dissolving any sense of seasons gone by. The trunk could just about fit two skinny girls, and standing there was to be inside something usually inaccessible, like touching another person's brain through their ear. It was a threshold into another world, of course, as all hollow trees are.

The hollow ash tree has remained there at the end of the farm the whole time and I am soon able to find it again. The grey-green lichen that covers the trunk is rough to the touch, like coral. Scars from when the fence-line ran right up against the tree, before Dad moved it, are slashed across the bark. Rusty barbed wire sticks out of the trunk in various places, from where the tree has absorbed the fence, like a person who's had a steel pin inserted into their leg to fix a break and a bolt or two sticks out above the flesh. Perhaps my memory is off, but the hollow ash tree looks no different at all from when I last climbed inside it, before I abandoned it and the whole business of tree climbing with an arrogant disregard for the wisdom of childhood.

Several hundred years old, my absence of a decade or so barely registers in the timescale of the tree. Its upper branches may have grown considerably, but its girth seems to have changed by only a few centimetres. These few centimetres are the distance I've moved from childhood. That's how close it is. The only really noticeable difference is that a large lower branch has fallen even lower and torn a hole in the side of the trunk, so that now I can peer inside. I pass an arm into the dark interior and feel the mix of leaf mulch, mud and rotting wood on the floor of the hollow. It feels like touching the mulch of memory itself.

Now, through this obsession with free flight, I am re-entering my body from the point of view of that boisterous prepubescent girl I found again, back on the farm, and took up into the sky. Some mornings, walking across the airfield to the launch point, I break into a run and do a couple of cartwheels along the way.

*

'Learning the secret of flight from a bird was a good deal like learning the secret of magic from a magician. After you know the trick and what to look for, you can see things you didn't notice when you did not know exactly what to look for.'

Orville Wright

I want to unlock the story of how people discovered unpowered flight and learned to soar like birds. Pilots bring to the club much-treasured books on the history of free flight to lend me, and I borrow others that I find in the clubhouse. And so my obsession is becoming a fascination. It is all enthralling: how free flight developed inside the larger history of how we got into the air; tales of pioneers, eccentrics and enthusiasts determined to get up into the sky and fly like a bird.

Leonardo da Vinci believed that, if he could discover the

secrets of the birds and find a way for humans to fly, he would gain 'glory eternal'. In sixteenth-century Italy, he spent hours watching black kites, skylarks and other birds, often buying caged birds in the markets of Florence just to set them free. Leonardo's fascination with flight was, according to one early biographer, 'the most tremendous, most obsessing, most tyrannical of his dreams'. His paintings are full of wings.

Da Vinci's notes and drawings became known long after his death as the *Codex on the Flight of Birds*, and he is one of the earliest thinkers to put pen to paper and pencil to drawing board in the hope of working out how humans could copy the birds. His design, which came to be called an 'ornithopter', was a machine with flapping wings, powered by the legs and arms of a man strapped inside using a series of ropes and pulleys.

Birds continued to be the blueprint for human flight well into the nineteenth century, the scientific age of invention, but flight remained a stubborn conundrum. By the late nineteenth century, inventors had successfully brought into being the telephone, electricity, telegraphy, sound recording, photography and primitive moving pictures, but birds refused to give up their secrets. It was an era that took on, with real determination, the awesome task of working out how a human could fly.

In his 1860s 'Letter on Flight', addressed 'to the whole world', Victor Hugo denounced the fascination with ballooning and prophesied the imminent birth of winged flight: 'the balloon has been judged, and found wanting . . .

To be torn from the ground like a dead leaf, to be swept along helplessly in a whirlwind, this is not true flying. And how do we achieve true flight? With wings!' Ships of the air would soon 'deliver mankind from the ancient tyranny of gravity,' he exclaimed, and man would become 'a thinking eagle with a soul.' Hugo predicted that the lighter-than-air balloon was the floating egg out of which the winged man-carrying bird would soon hatch. And when that day came, 'the old Gordian knot of gravity will finally be untied,' and there would be a 'brisk flinging open of the ancient cage door of history, a flooding in of light.'

Many of the designs for flying apparatus, prototype flying models and full-size flying machines, by enthusiastic inventors who shared Hugo's vision of the future, continued to be directly inspired by the ornithopter design. Jacob Degan of Vienna designed an ornithopter; he drew a man in a suit standing inside a square frame with arched wings sprouting from his shoulders. He was to be carried aloft by balloon and then released into the air. A Frenchman named Letur went out and gave his invention a try; he built an elaborate apparatus that was a mix of a flapping-winged ornithopter and a primitive parachute, which he intended to launch from beneath a hot-air balloon. He became tangled in trees after lift-off and was killed. A Belgian named De Groof followed suit, but he fell to his death in 1874. The ornithopter design wasn't proving very successful.

There were several prototype flying machines on display at the 1868 Crystal Palace exhibition in London, which

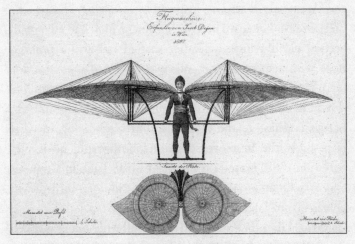

Engraving of Jacob Degen's ornithopter design, 1807.

included the first air show in history. It was a futuristic, rather fantastical show, because none of the exhibits had actually flown. Some had been tried and failed to get airborne, others were designs that had yet to be tested. And so, decades before successful human flying machines were invented, prototype flying machines, stepping right out of Jules Verne's aerial science-fiction adventure stories, were on display. Some were cobbled-together hybrids: a mix of birds, boats, horse carriages and balloons. One of the designs on show was for a giant mechanical bird with a man sitting inside it – a Trojan raptor.

The turning point came when people began to take their inspiration from soaring birds and to design machines with fixed (rather than flapping) wings. A French sea captain called Jean-Marie Le Bris built a glider that he called the 'Artificial Albatross', inspired by a soaring albatross he had observed at sea. The contraption, which had two giant arched cloth wings, a feather-shaped tail and a pointed nose with a spike on the end, was mounted on a wooden farm cart with huge wheels for take-off. Le Bris trundled downhill on the cart and then launched briefly into the air, before crashing to the ground and breaking a leg. In what is possibly the first ever aviation photograph, he is pictured, in 1868, seated on the giant bird's back in a top hat and coachman's coat, as if he were riding a bird-drawn chariot from fairy tales of old.

Otto Lilienthal designed and built lightweight fixed wings that rested on his shoulders and attached to his body with a harness. His designs were inspired by the storks he'd watched soaring over his village in Germany when he was a child. An engineer by trade, he poured all his finances and energy into his flying experiments and made almost 2,000 descending flights in home-made gliders. He was a scientist, engineer and naturalist, and his scrupulous studies of birds led him to believe that only a curved or cambered wing could produce lift. From 1885 to 1896, he thrilled people across the world as tales spread of his adventures leaping from the top of a home-made fifty-foot hill, strapped into elegant waxed-cloth and willow-wood wings. He tried numerous different designs: one was a two-tiered biplane; another looked like a soaring eagle, with large wings that had fingered tips, like a raptor's primary feathers. His gliders had no controls, so he had to use his body weight to try to counter currents and

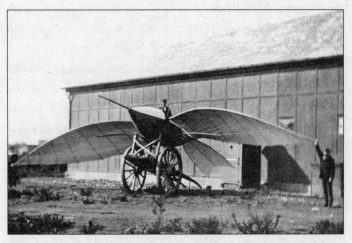

Jean-Marie Le Bris in the cockpit of his flying machine
Albatros II, 1868.

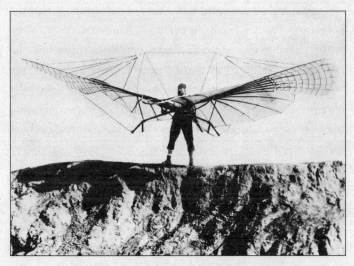

Otto Lilienthal's early gliding trials *c.*1891.

manoeuvre through the air. He would throw his legs energetically from one side to the other to counter gusts of fickle and unpredictable wind.

Photos of Lilienthal were printed in the international press, and across the world he became known as the 'Glider King', the first celebrity aviator, though fellow engineers working on heavily financed projects to develop steam-powered flying machines (none of which would ever fly) dismissed him as a 'flying squirrel'. A visiting American journalist who witnessed the extraordinary spectacle of Lilienthal leaping from his hill was struck by the sounds his flying contraption made. The waxed-cotton cloth spread over the willow-wood struts as tight as a drum meant the wings reverberated if you touched them. Flying above the head of the beguiled journalist, the apparatus made a strange noise as the wind whistled over its bracing chords, becoming a weird, man-carrying aeolian harp.

In possibly the world's first ever description of the rapture of gliding, Lilienthal wrote of 'the indescribable beauty and gentle sensation of gliding along over the expanse of sunlit mountain-slopes' that 'serves merely to increase one's ardour' for flying. 'No one can realize how substantial the air is until he feels its supporting power beneath him. It inspires confidence.'

In the summer of 1896, Lilienthal took off in a fresh wind, hit a strong gust and his wing was forced into a stall. He tumbled to the ground and broke his back. He died a few hours later.

News of Lilienthal's tragic death travelled across the

Atlantic to Dayton, Ohio, and to two brothers called Orville and Wilbur Wright, who ran a bicycle business. They had followed Lilienthal's flying experiments and were inspired to continue his work of exploring the realm of the birds, but they quickly realized that it was necessary to develop a means of control in the air. 'The wings should move, not the man,' wrote Octave Chanute, an aviation enthusiast and inventor who corresponded with the Wrights.

The Wrights' gliding achievements and contributions to the development of free flight are often hidden inside the larger story of their successful invention of controlled powered flight, but before they could add an engine to power an aircraft, the Wrights knew they had to fully understand how a wing worked and how it could be manoeuvred through the air.

Initially, they experimented with tethered man-carrying kites as a way of studying, close up, the ways in which a wing responds to the air. In 1900, they built a fabric and pine 'Kite Flyer' that they flew on the sands of Kitty Hawk, North Carolina, taking turns to ride it. 'If the plan will enable me to remain in the air for practice by hours instead of by the second,' wrote Wilbur, 'I hope to acquire skills sufficient to overcome the difficulties inherent in flight.'

The Kite Flyer was a simple design of two cloth-and-pine wings, one on top of the other, with a line of struts holding them together. It looked a bit like a flying box, and bucked like a bronco in the wind, but it gave the brothers useful information about flying. One day, at the end of the summer, the Kite Flyer was left unguarded on the ground for a moment, and a gust took it into the air and smashed it back on to the sand. The brothers went back to Ohio for the winter, abandoning what remained of their incredible experiment, and a local family used the sateen fabric to make dresses for their daughters.

After their experiments with tethered man-carrying kites, the Wrights spent a number of years flying untethered gliders on the same sands. These were two-tiered biplanes made of cloth and wood, with various kinds of tail and rudder designs. Orville or Wilbur would lie facedown in the middle of the lower wing to pilot the glider, and the other brother and a friend would stabilize the wings while it was launched from a primitive downhill ramp. They flew over 1,000 glider flights, some for a distance of as much as 600 feet; most were forms of gradual descent down a hill, but occasionally the glider would maintain its height in the slope wind. It stayed up, even if it didn't *rise* up. Their skill and control got so fine that they were able, like the buzzards they observed, to hover in one spot, into wind, to hang almost motionless in the air. The Wright brothers were the first to experience controlled ridge soaring.

From observations of soaring birds riding on upwelling currents of air, the Wrights were convinced that it might be possible to ascend on thermals and ridge winds without an engine. As early as 1901, Wilbur wrote, 'when gliding operators have attained greater skill, they can, with com-

parative safety, maintain themselves in the air for hours at
a time in this way, and thus by constant practice so increase
their knowledge and skill that they can rise into the higher
air and search out the currents which enable the soaring
birds to transport themselves to any desired point by first
rising in a circle and then sailing off'.

I'm excited to see that, before the invention of powered
flight, the Wrights already understood the key distinction
between gliding and soaring, and intuited that it might
be possible to sail on the wind, like birds. The term 'glider',
I realize, is in some ways misleading, because free flight,
unlike sky diving and wing-suit flying, which are forms
of elegant descent, is all about staying up and ascending,
soaring higher and higher. The Wrights understood that
potential.

The Wrights triumphed at inventing sustained powered
flight in 1903, and the world became entranced. But the
brothers quietly kept alive their fascination with gliding.
In 1911, Orville returned to Kill Devil Hills in North
Carolina, where they had flown many of their experimental machines, to test a new stability control system.
Orville abandoned the test and decided instead to do
some gliding. On one flight, he remained aloft on the wind
for nine minutes, a world soaring record that would stand
until 1921.

At this point, the histories of powered and unpowered
flight largely separate to branch in different directions,
and, in the rush of excitement at the birth of powered
flight, unpowered flying was almost forgotten. But small

pockets of enthusiasm for gliding remained. The desire to soar like a bird continued to fuel some eccentrics, including French-born naturalized Englishman Jose Weiss, a landscape painter and aviation enthusiast who was inspired by the beauty of Lilienthal's gliders. In 1909, Weiss built a glider with swept back, swallow-shaped wings spanning twenty-six feet, which he flew from the Sussex Downs, near Arundel. Weiss knew it would be possible to soar on up currents from watching soaring birds on hilltops and cliff tops, but it was his assistant, a young railway engineer called Eric Gordon-England, who learned to pilot Weiss's glider very well, to feel the up currents with his body and manoeuvre the glider in contact with the air to stay aloft for several minutes at a time.

In 1909, Gordon-England managed a flight in Weiss's swallow-shaped glider that would later be considered the moment real gliding was born: he travelled almost a mile forward and, most importantly, he rose in lift. He went up! He ascended! This was a key turning point in the development of free flight, and led to a group of enthusiasts, including Weiss and Gordon-England, banding together in 1912 to form the first British soaring club – the Amberley Aviation Society. Suddenly, the sky could take you places.

While Weiss was developing his glider, a German architect called Friedrich Harth was working on his design for what would become the first practical, stable (crucially, the glider had a tail, unlike Weiss's) free-flight aircraft. Harth was determined to design something that would fly without an engine, and, before the outbreak of the war, he made several flights and managed to stay aloft in ridge lift for three minutes.

But then the Great War engulfed the world, crushing those adventures and killing many of the young men who had enjoyed them. If the war decimated the population of potential pilots, though, the post-war context created the very conditions for unpowered flight to properly develop.

By the end of the First World War, the aeroplane was understood to be a weapon and, under the conditions of the Treaty of Versailles, Germany was prohibited from re-arming and from building an air force. But this didn't stop them from building unpowered gliders. Enthusiasm and engineering know-how continued to thrive in Germany and groups began to meet regularly to fly in home-made gliders. As designs and piloting expertise grew, flights became longer.

Energy was particularly centred at the Wasserkuppe, the highest peak of the Rhön Mountains, where, in 1921, Wilhelm Leusch was pulled up into the powerful rising air current of a cumulonimbus monster. Spectators watched from the ground in horror as his wings crumpled to pieces and the shattered plane and its pilot tumbled to earth. But Leusch's tragic flight showed that gliders could find enormous amounts of energetic lift in the thermals beneath clouds. Pilots started to explore thermal soaring, moving away from the apron strings of ridge lift produced over hills. It was extremely dangerous and several more pilots died, but, in 1929, a German pilot succeeded in flying eighty-five miles.

The discovery of thermal lift in Germany inspired the gliding movement across the world. In 1930, the U.S. held its first soaring meeting in Elmira, New York, and Wolf Hirth, a daredevil pioneer glider pilot from the Wasser-kuppe, travelled to the States for the meeting. Hirth had lost a leg in a motorbike accident (he had the fibula from his amputated leg made into a cigarette holder), so he flew with a wooden prosthetic controlling the rudder pedal. Hirth knew he should follow the birds to fly in invisible thermals and later wrote, 'I caught sight of two soaring birds wheeling and gaining height rapidly. They showed me where I could find further lift.' He also wrote, 'I felt com-pletely identified with my sailplane and at that moment would not have exchanged it for the fastest and most expensive power plane in the world.'

On the same trip, Hirth flew from a quay on the Hudson River, over the city of New York, maintaining his height of 1,000 feet by soaring in the thermals and ridge lift created by the buildings. Crowds gathered to watch and the traffic on Broadway was brought to a standstill. Needless to say, the authorities were not impressed.

Back in Germany, the story of free flight was taking on a darker hue. Unbeknownst to the rest of the world, the popular gliding movement in Germany was training what would later become the core pilots of the Luftwaffe. The German air force was being formed in defiance of the Treaty of Versailles and many of its pilots were being trained to fly in gliders. In 1938, a captain in the Luftwaffe gained a world altitude record when he flew in a glider to

21,400 feet. It's a chilling thought; the dream of soaring like an albatross was being twisted by history.

With the outbreak of the Second World War, a war that would be decisively played out in the skies, gliding became a tool in the armoury on all sides.

The first ever glider-borne assault was in May 1940, when the Germans successfully invaded the supposedly impenetrable Belgian fortress of Eben-Emael. The plan was designed by Hitler and saw ten gliders deliver troops, at sunrise, to the inner sanctum of the fort and on to nearby strategically placed bridges. Once the gliders had been towed up and had made their descent and landed, they were abandoned. The Germans also invaded Crete in 1941, delivering troops in silent gliders flown on tow behind power planes.

The Allies formed glider regiments too. U.S. war correspondent Walter Cronkite was commissioned into a glider regiment and was flown into the aerial invasion of Holland, in 1944. The experience made a deep impression on the young journalist: 'gliders were landing around us . . . But others came tumbling out of the sky. Two collided almost above us and a jeep and a howitzer, and soldiers, came crashing down. A C-47 came in low overhead, streaming smoke and exploded in the woods just beyond. Another glider came straight down and plowed into the soft earth like an artillery shell. The field was scattered with gliders on their noses, on their sides, on their backs. It was a scene from hell'.

Gliders were also widely used in the Allied invasion of

Normandy. Towed over the Channel in the dark and released to descend to the ground, pilots were horrified when they realized that the Germans, predicting the aerial invasion in gliders, had littered the ground with posts that made landing almost impossible. It was carnage.

One wartime glider, the 'Colditz Cock', became famous despite the fact that it never flew. In the spring of 1945, a group of twelve Allied prisoners of war, held in Colditz Castle, designed and built a glider from pieces of wooden furniture and bedclothes stolen from the castle. Led by Bill Goldfinch and Jack Best, they worked on a machine based on what they read in a book on aircraft design from the castle library. The wing spars were fashioned from floorboards and the ribs from bed slats. The control cables were electrical wires taken from the castle, and they used millet to make the glue to seal the bedclothes that covered the glider's wooden structure. They built it in the attic above the castle chapel, hidden behind a false wall. The plan was to launch it from the rooftop on a runway of tables, to fly over the River Mulde during an air-raid blackout. But the war ended and the prisoners were released before they had a chance to escape, though I'm sure the idea of an aerial departure must have kept their spirits up.

Once the war was over, the gliding movement, like everything else, was in tatters. But many free-flight enthusiasts from the 1930s, on both sides of the war, had survived, and they soon rekindled their passion for free flying, built aircraft and formed associations and clubs. By the 1950s, an international gliding movement across the world, though small, was full of brave enthusiasts who continued to push the boundaries of what it was thought possible to do in an unpowered aircraft, flying ever higher, further and for longer, exploring the energy in the sky. While powered flight grew into commercial air travel and developed the jet engine, free flight, now released from its association with war, held fast to the spirit that had fuelled the early pioneers of flight and the dream of soaring like a bird.

Chapter Seven

Have We Fallen Off the Edge of Wonder?

'Real flight and dreams of flight go together. Both are part of the same movement. Not A before B, but all together.'

Thomas Pynchon

In my passion for flying, I see something of the enthusiasm with which both powered and unpowered flight were greeted in the early twentieth century, which our wider culture has now largely lost or abandoned. What's happened to our relationship with human flight? At any one moment, a British Airways pilot told me, there are approximately 500,000 people, across the planet, who are airborne. Flying is global, commonplace; we've become dependent on air travel and it's become banal. 'Today, flying means being hurled into an overcrowded aluminium tube at 40,000ft with your knees around your ears,' wrote Stuart Jeffries in the *Guardian*.

That article was published in spring 2010, when the unpronounceable Icelandic volcano Eyjafjallajökull erupted, grounding all flights across the Western world for six days.

Not since the Second World War had the U.K. experienced such an extensive flight ban. Trade was at a standstill, millions of people were stranded, vegetables bound for airfreight were rotting, cut flowers were wilting in Kenya, and medicines and aid packages were dangerously delayed. But, despite all this, the U.K. celebrated.

In his article, published a few days into the flight ban, Jeffries asked if readers were enjoying the clear skies. It seemed that many people were. On Saturday, 17 April, a blog post read, 'This morning I took the dog for a walk and for a while I couldn't quite put my finger on what was different . . . Not just clear of clouds but clear of vapour trails. I was looking at the sky as it must have been 100 years ago. This had a profound impact on me. No noise. The air is completely free of even high level distant aircraft noise and I never realised just how pervasive the noise has been. Today is a beautiful day. We have Eyjafjallajoekull (sic) the Icelandic Volcano to thank for this.'

Jeffries noted how, without the noise of jet engines, he was able to savour the birdsong in London. 'Enjoy it while it lasts,' an elderly gentleman advised him.

At the beginning of the twenty-first century, taking to the skies has, for most people, become associated with discomfort, light entertainment, bad novels, duty-free cigarettes and alcohol, and bland shopping-mall airports, or with terrorism, military violence, air and noise pollution, climate change and, for some, fear of catastrophic crashes. 'You define a good flight by negatives,' wrote travel writer Paul Theroux: 'you didn't get hijacked, you didn't crash, you didn't throw up, you weren't late, you weren't nauseated by the food. So you are grateful.'

Only a hundred years after we first took to the sky, we seem to have already fallen out of love. But how different things were at the beginning of the twentieth century. The birth of human flight was greeted with elation, shock, disbelief. It seemed to be a miracle – one which many learned men had predicted would be impossible. It was a profoundly emotional response that reflected the deep and ancient human yearning to fly, a species-wide longing, a Promethean desire to make gods of ourselves.

In 1910, a plane flew over Chicago for the first time, attracting a crowd estimated at over a million. A priest was amongst the spectators and wrote afterwards, 'never have I seen such a look of wonder in the faces of the multitude. From the grey-haired man to the child, everyone seemed to feel that it was a new day in their lives.' A Mary M. Parker wrote, 'We bowed our heads before the mystery of it and then lifted our eyes with a new feeling in our souls that seemed to link us all, and hope sprang eternal for the great new future of the world.' We were at last able to explore what had seemed an inaccessible realm, a place into which we had projected our gods and devils. People fell in love with flying, with the very idea of it.

There was something evangelical about the cause of human flight in its early decades. A new age was upon us – an 'air age' – and it would usher in the brave new world of the future. It would be one of reform, peace and social improvement. Soon, everybody would fly and a kind of democracy in the sky would appear. Evangelists of flight predicted that there would be aerial sanatoriums, health spas in the sky (because altitude was thought to be good for you). 'Up, up into the pure microbeless air,' cried one enthusiast, 'the sick and suffering will be carried and nursed back to health in private air sanatoria and state and municipal air hospitals.' There would be an aeroplane in every garage and people would commute to work from green remote suburbs to city centres in their flying cars. In the Chicago World's Fair of 1933, an exhibit called 'The Home of Tomorrow' was complete with a plane port for a small aeroplane. This was the promise of aviation, the 'Winged Gospel'.

On the outer fringes of this enthusiasm, I discover some strange ideas. Montagu, Lord Norman (1871–1950) was an establishment figure, educated at Eton and Cambridge before becoming an officer in the army, and later Governor of the Bank of England, between 1920 and 1944. Lord Norman had rather eccentric interests in the occult and the paranormal, and he regularly had ecstatic and highly realistic flying dreams, in which he would soar and weave through the sky. He'd wake convinced that there must be some reality to these extraordinary dreams, and he couldn't understand how and why flying, uncommon and strange to the waking world, became for him and others such a natural feature of sleep.

He concluded that the only reasonable explanation for his flying dreams was that they were an atavistic memory echo of a time when humans could fly. His version of the expulsion of Adam and Eve from the Garden of Eden after the Fall was rewritten as the idea that we once were able to fly, but lost the knowledge. We fell back to earth.

Lord Norman shared his odd theories with Air Chief Marshal Lord Dowding (1882–1970), who was Air Officer Commanding R.A.F. Fighter Command during the Battle of Britain. Lord Dowding thought there might be something in Lord Norman's idea. He thought it possible that there was a 'root race' of 'pre-Adamite' humans who could levitate and fly.

Lords Norman and Dowding weren't the first or only people to speculate about the possibility that humans flew in the past. In the eighteenth century, the Italian natural philosopher Tiberius Cavallo wondered if the idea of human flight 'might be the result of pure imagination – or perhaps an art which was lost.' More recently, the Peruvian Nazca Lines have been cited by some as evidence that humans must have had some means of flying. For how, so the idea goes, could the ancient Peruvians have designed and fashioned such enormous coherent landscape drawings of spiders, humming birds, monkeys and lizards? And how could they have witnessed them, once they were finished, other than by taking to the air?

Eccentric ideas about the future of human flight surfaced during the era of the Winged Gospel too. Alfred Lawson was an influential American aviation publisher and aeroplane designer, who designed one of the first passenger airliners in 1919: a twenty-six seater. He was an enthusiastic private pilot, who flew a small plane between his home and office. In an article in an aviation journal, he prophesied that, by AD 3000, pilots would never land, and, by the year 10000, they would have evolved into a distinctive subspecies of human. 'Altiman' would live permanently in the sky, able to grow food in the upper air and control the weather. According to Lawson, Altiman wouldn't be able to come back down to earth because his biology would have evolved to live at altitude. Ground men would live like crabs on the bottom of the atmospheric ocean, while Altiman would swim unaided in the air above.

Other people also predicted the evolution of a flying human being. Charlotte Perkins Gilman, American feminist and experimental writer, suggested, in the same era, that an 'aerial person' would evolve. In an article in *Harpers* called 'When We Fly', she predicted that the new aerial human would metamorphose out of the 'earthy' human, as the butterfly emerges from the caterpillar. The flying machine was the pupa out of which the flying aerial person would eventually hatch.

The magnificent discovery of human flight, combined with the age-old mystery of persistent and realistic flying dreams, had clearly turned some people's heads. But these eccentric ideas touch on something that I have come to know to be true, while learning to fly: how natural it feels to be in the air. I feel at home, up there. As instructions swirl inside my head and the horizon twists and slips across the canopy as we circle inside a thermal, flying nevertheless feels like I'm *re*learning something I've forgotten. Soaring already has the quality of a well-loved and familiar memory.

In becoming possessed by free flight, I'm participating in an old story – the same one that took hold of many people's imaginations in the first half of the twentieth century. If powered flight has been tainted by commercial air travel, in the subculture of free flight in which I'm immersed, the passion for flying is kept truly alive; there's no disillusionment here. Milling about in the clubhouse, if anyone hears the sound of a low-flying engine, they rush to the window to see what it is. A mountain-rescue helicopter, a small propeller plane, a fighter jet practising manoeuvres in these hills – it doesn't matter; heads look up with enthusiasm, as they did for the first decades of human flight, when seeing a plane in the air was a marvel. It's still marvellous here.

*

One of the icons of the golden age of flight was the aviatrix. At the beginning of the twentieth century, she was a symbol of the New Woman's freedom to ride bicycles, vote, smoke cigarettes, use contraceptives, go to university, earn money and own property. I'm delighted to come across these exciting female pilots from history. The gliding club is sadly low on female members and I've found myself wondering why. But I can turn to history to discover what role women pilots played in the development of unpowered flight.

On one of my trawls through the aviation sections of

second-hand bookshops in Hay-on-Wye, a twenty-minute drive from the airfield, I come across a large coffee-table book full of gorgeous black-and-white photographs of women aviators looking unexpectedly feminine in their leather and sheepskin jackets, flying suits and goggles. Flying challenged the accepted norms of what women could wear, and the 1920s flying flapper looked fantastic in her bright lipstick and black eye make-up, jodhpurs, knee-high leather boots, white shirts and fetching silk scarves.

'Flying is the best possible thing for women,' wrote the Frenchwoman Elise Deroche, the first woman to fly solo in an aeroplane.

'Flying is the only real freedom,' wrote Louise Thaden, an early American pilot.

'Flying is more exciting than love,' asserted Germany's Thea Rasche, another 1920s aviatrix.

'Fear is a tonic and danger something of a stimulant,' wrote Mary Heath, after her pioneering solo flight from Cape Town to London in 1928.

I am pleased to discover that women also took to the skies without an engine in between the wars. One particular female glider pilot stands out as a key pioneer of free flight, both before and after the war. But I find her story troubling.

Hanna Reitsch was a diminutive glider pilot who showed exceptional flying skill in 1930s Germany. She had wanted to fly like a bird since her childhood, took gliding lessons while still in high school, and showed real talent and courage; her male classmates nicknamed her 'Stratosphere'. She was so tiny that she had a glider tailor-made to suit her miniature stature, and in it she went on to establish numerous endurance, distance and altitude gliding world records before the war, including being the first woman to fly across the Alps.

Reitsch was also a dedicated Nazi. She became a flying instructor for the Flieger-Hitlerjugend, the Flying Hitler Youth. She also performed as a flying stunt double in Nazi propaganda movies before the war. In 1934, she joined a German gliding expedition to South America to study thermal conditions. She was accompanied by fellow German pilots Peter Riedel, Heini Dittmar and Wolf Hirth, the one-legged glider pilot who had flown over New York City. In Argentina, Reitsch watched vultures soaring on giant wings. She circled up in thermals with a dozen or so birds, flying right up close to them: 'we found it possible to fly over wide stretches of lonely plain and forest, which we would never have been able to do without the aid of our reliable "pilots".' She was so taken with the aerial guides that she had four caught and brought back to Germany, where she planned to use them to guide her to thermals. But, back in Germany, the birds refused to leave their enclosure until they were shooed out, and even then they merely flopped up into a tree. One bird disappeared and was later seen walking in the street in Heidelberg. Realizing that the experiment had failed, Reitsch gave the other three to Frankfurt zoo.

At less than five feet tall, Reitsch was still an imposing figure in German aviation during the Second World
War, having somehow escaped the restrictions brought in
by the Nazis on the possible occupations for women outside the home. Her flying skills were widely recognized
and she became a test pilot for the Luftwaffe, trying out a
large range of fighters and bombers, and troop-carrying
gliders. She had reached that point predicted by Wilbur
Wright: 'When she flew,' said a colonel in the Luftwaffe,
'it was like anyone else going for a walk – she had mas-
tered the medium.' She was the first woman to receive the
Pilot/Observer Badge in Gold with Diamonds, which was
awarded personally by Göring. Her specially made medal
was in the form of a brooch.

Such was her lack of fear and her commitment and
patriotism that, towards the end of the war, when the
possibility of a German victory looked bleak, she came up
with a diabolical scheme: to develop a suicide-bombing
unit of pilots, Operation Suicide. This unit would undertake suicide missions in Britain and against the Allies on
land and sea, flying glider-bombs into key targets. The idea
of willingly sacrificing pilots was not well received by the
Luftwaffe, but, in 1944, Reitsch recruited seventy pilots,
including some women, to carry out the suicide missions.
Luckily, the Allied D-Day landings in Normandy scup-
pered these horrific plans and they were never carried out.

At the end of the war, Reitsch was captured and inter-
rogated briefly, but she wasn't charged with war crimes,
and so, from the 1950s onwards, she continued to pursue

her passion for gliding, setting new world records, winning competitions and travelling abroad to promote free flight. In 1959, the German government sent her to India as a gliding ambassador. A jet fighter had crashed into a hangar at the gliding centre in Delhi, destroying all their aircraft, and Germany was giving the club a new glider and sending Reitsch to deliver it. She flew an aerobatics display over Delhi for an astonished crowd below, and followed it with a joyful two-hour flight with the former Indian Prime Minister, Jawaharlal Nehru. How curious it is to think of the Nazi test-pilot Valkyrie soaring with the first Prime Minister of newly independent India.

Reitsch went on to court more political controversy when, in the 1960s, she travelled to Ghana, where she set up the first African gliding school with the support of the dictator Nkrumah, with whom she was said to be close. Struggling to set up the school in a dusty cattle pasture, rented from a local chief, who was paid in gin, she demanded funds from the government of Ghana for facilities, not acknowledging that the impoverished country might have more important things to fund than a flying school. Characteristically obsessive and culturally insensitive, she cut down a tree without adherence to the correct customs and rituals, much to the horror of locals. She escaped Ghana in 1966, in disguise, after the coup d'état that deposed Nkrumah, joining him briefly in Guinea before heading back to Germany.

Reitsch gained her fortieth gliding record at the age of sixty-seven, in April 1979, and died four months later under suspicious circumstances. Rumours, now heavily disputed, circulated that Reitsch took the cyanide pill she had been given by Hitler during the war.

I find the story of Reitsch's life disquieting. I understand her passion for gliding, but it seems to have blinded her to humanity on the ground. Many pilots admire her flying skills and appreciate her extraordinary enthusiasm for free flight, but her commitment to the Nazi project and her appetite for political controversy cast a shadow over her. There was clearly a fanatical dimension to her character. What bothers me most about her is the possibility that her commitment to free flight, something I felt I understood, came somehow from the same dark place in her mind that inspired her commitment to Hitler, to the Nazis and to the idea of Operation Suicide. To me, there was something diabolical in Reitsch's fearlessness, something that should have been beautiful, but became twisted.

But I discover some less troubling female heroines of the free-flight movement as well. World-famous British aviatrix Amy Johnson, the first woman to fly from the U.K. to Australia in a power plane, also enjoyed gliding and flew at the Long Mynd in Shropshire in the 1930s. Gliding was popular in Poland, and the brilliantly named Wanda Modlibonka stayed aloft, in 1937, for a record-breaking twenty-four hours. In Russia, Olga Klepikova achieved what some pilots now regard as a rather suspiciously spectacular world distance record in July 1939, one month before the outbreak of the Second World War (it has been suggested that the claim was Soviet propaganda).

Klepikova was said to have flown 465 miles (749 kilo-metres) in a bright red glider, from Moscow to Stalingrad – almost twice the distance record at the time and one that remained unbroken until 1951.

And a young British army officer's wife and society journalist with aspirations to write romantic novels took up gliding in the 1930s. Discussing flying with two R.A.F. officer friends in 1931, Barbara Cartland came up with the idea of launching gliders with towplanes and using them to deliver goods, and, true to her word, later that year, she flew a glider 200 miles on tow to deliver the post. Although the Germans had already thought of it, Cartland also came up with the idea of delivering troops by glider. In 1984, she was awarded the Bishop Wright Air Industry Award for her contribution to aviation. History doesn't record whether or not her flying suit was pink.

Another star woman glider of the 1930s was Joan Meakin. She was determined to fly after she read *Peter Pan* as a child, and she learned to fly in Germany, at the Wasserkuppe, and towed her new glider all the way from Germany to England. In 1934, Meakin became the first woman to cross the English Channel by a glider on tow, looping several times before she came in to land in France. On landing, after a bumpy ride over the sea, she was inter-viewed for Pathé News and said that gliding was 'safer than playing hockey'. She married Ronald Price, a wing walker with Alan Cobham's Flying Circus, and joined the troupe as the 'Titian-haired' glider aerobatics aviatrix. They travelled the country in the early 1930s like barnstormers, giving air displays at airfields and in farmers' fields to a fascinated public, many of whom had never seen an aeroplane before, let alone a young red-headed woman piloting a giant wooden bird without an engine, tumbling, falling, rising and looping through the air. She would be towed up to several thousand feet, where she would release and then perform numerous loop-the-loops and other manoeuvres, before landing back in the field from which she had taken off. Her record was eighteen consecutive loops. I can't imagine arcing through the air so many times in a row, the G-force pressing in and receding, over and over again, the world turning and turning.

*

And now it's my turn. It's a wet August day and Bo and I have been in the air for just over an hour. There are curtains of rain clouds floating over the River Wye, creating rainbows low to the ground. We are in a steep banking turn, flying at about fifty knots, ascending in a thermal at six knots, and I am filled with elation – it's sending me into a kind of focused trance.

As we head back towards the airfield, Bo whistles behind me softly. He goes quiet for a moment or two and then asks, 'Shall we do a loop?'

'What? Well, OK,' I reply tentatively.

'Watch the speed and tell me when we hit ninety knots,' he says, kindly including me in the manoeuvre. He pushes the stick forward a touch, our nose drops and we immediately pick up speed. The air howls over the wings and the fuselage, getting louder as we speed up; it is almost deafening. I watch the needle on the speedometer swing around to the right.

'Ninety!' I shout, and Bo gently pulls the stick back. Our nose begins to rise, the horizon starts to fall away and I feel the G-force dig into me, pushing me back into my parachute and seat. My head presses against the rest and I can't move it. Suddenly, all I see is blue, and I'm pinned back into my seat by the sky itself. We're flying almost vertically upwards, the sun passes by, we tip backwards and then we're upside down. It's strange to see fields suspended in space, woodland dangling from above; the hills look like the underneath of hammocks with people asleep in them. I'm upside down and it feels right to have the sky underneath me, a blue anchor. I have been turned on my head.

As we loop back, the G-force gradually recedes and I can move my head again. I let out a long laugh as we dip towards the end of the circle and flatten out, earth beneath, sky above. The roar of the air dies down as we slow to fifty knots and fly horizontally towards the airfield. I land, still chuckling, with a sense of having been loosened and turned inside out as well as upside down.

*

In the past few weeks, I've let go of any attempt to control risk. Instead, I relax into it, am hardly aware of any risk at all, in fact. Any fear has completely disappeared. Bo notices this and thinks I am ready to work on an important aspect of flying: learning what to do when things go wrong. My fearlessness comes to the fore when we start to practise stalls and spins, high in the sky.

'Most pilots,' says Bo, 'are a little bit anxious about doing stalls and spins. For many students, it's one of the most frightening aspects of learning to fly.' He explains further: the 'angle of attack' is the angle at which the wing meets the air flowing over and under it to create lift. Increasing the angle of attack by lifting the nose will mean that eventually the glider reaches a point where the air is no longer flowing over and under the wings sufficiently to create lift. Then you're in a stall. Each aircraft design has a different point at which it stalls, so you must come to learn the boundaries of your particular glider. 'Most importantly,' says Bo, 'you must learn to recognize the feel of an imminent stall.'

When the glider reaches the point of stall and the wings stop flying, the heaviest part of the glider, the nose, falls forward and you head for the ground. It's tempting to pull hard back on the stick to raise the nose, but the stick will be totally ineffectual if you do that. You must move the stick to the neutral position, somewhere near the middle, pause for a second and then slowly pull it back to restore the normal angle of attack, and you are flying again. That's recovering from a straight stall.

A spin is when one wing stalls before the other; you stall and nosedive *and* spiral, spinning downwards like a falling autumn leaf. A spin was known as a 'death spiral' during the First World War because it killed so many pilots who didn't understand stalling and spinning sufficiently. To get out of a stalling spin, you need to do a series of specific manoeuvres quickly and decisively. First, press fully down on the rudder pedal of the opposite direction to which you are spinning, then neutralize the stick, neutralize the rudder and, finally, pull the stick back to restore normal flying attitude.

It's not easy to put a glider into a stall and spin; they're designed to avoid them, but Bo says that I need to know how to recognize the signs – the juddering of the wings, the nose high on the horizon, the poor response of the controls and reduced noise as the flying speed slows – and what to do to get out of it in the unlikely event that it does happen. There are no instruments that can help if you get into a stall or spin situation. You have to feel it, and react immediately. The stall and spin are both very dangerous if they happen close to the ground. 'You're dead, probably,' says Bo.

We practise stalls and spins at altitude to ensure there's enough space to recover. I have my instruments hidden. It's probably more unnerving to be able to see them, to be able to watch the altimeter winding down as we head for the ground. Having completed our checks, Bo tells me to gently pull back on the stick and raise the nose. I pull back; the nose rears up. Bo tells me to be more gentle, go more slowly, using smaller movements on the controls; I follow his instruction, pulling back more gently. The sound of the rushing air quietens as we slow and as the nose points up into the sky. Soon, I can see nothing but blue out of the cockpit. Then we stall. The nose drops and we're heading straight for the ground, the air howling loudly again, my stomach lurching as we dive downwards.

'Stick to neutral,' I hear from the back, and Bo is on the controls with me. His movements are decisive and calm. 'Now, gently pull the stick back.' We begin to fly normally again.

We do it again, then again, then again, until eventually we've lost height and must head back to the airfield. I'm surprised to find that I enjoy the sensation of sudden quiet, followed by a pause, before tipping forward and rushing towards the ground; it's thrilling, and I look forward to doing it again. I'm finding it hard to remember the exact order of the moves to recover from a stall, so I'll need to practise it a lot, and I relish the thought of it.

A few days later, we progress to practising spin stalls. We stall, fall sideways, and then we're spinning around and around with the nose facing directly down towards the ground. I look down between my knees at the green fields 4,000 feet below. They seem to rotate around us. As we continue to spin, Bo talks through the procedure: 'Full and opposite rudder, stick to neutral, neutralize the rudder, and pull back on the stick.' I accompany him on the controls to follow the set of moves, and we pull up out of the free fall and all is well.

I feel my pulse as we bump and jolt in a bit of turbulence after recovering from the spin. My heart rate remains slow and steady. *Thump, thump, thump*, it goes, unresponsive. I've the curiously numb feeling of having moved beyond fear. I'm right on the edge of myself, where I don't feel afraid. I wonder where this strange fearlessness will lead.

*

I begin to ask people about their attitude to risk and what frightens them. The responses are so subjective.

John Coward tells me he fears confined spaces. If he accidentally wraps himself up in his bed sheet at night, he wakes in terror. 'That's really frightening,' he says, and I picture his heart pumping slow and steady as he comes in to land in the pitch dark at a hundred miles per hour on a moving aircraft carrier surrounded by a black sea.

I tell some gliding friends that I am thinking of doing a skydive and they suck in air around their teeth. 'Oh, I wouldn't do that.'

Watching trails of children on horseback passing by the entrance to the airfield, some pilots say they fear being at the mercy of an unpredictable animal. Bikers say they'd never fly without an engine. Glider pilots say they feel safer in an unpowered plane than in a powered plane; the sky, they point out, won't suddenly stop working. People who drive at ninety miles an hour on the motorway say they wouldn't go gliding or horse riding or motorbiking. Some of the same people fear going on a transatlantic jet, even though it's far safer. We twist the knowledge we have of the world around to suit us.

Research has shown that reliable statistics have little impact on people's subjective risk assessment. Our blurry brains edit out information we don't want to include and magnify whatever fits our preferred picture of what's risky and frightening and what isn't.

Bo admits to me that many of his fellow pilots say you're more likely to have a dangerous accident driving to a flying club than during gliding itself. 'But it's not true,' he says. 'I've known so many people to die gliding, at least ten, and I don't know anyone who has died in a traffic accident.'

I'm not sure how I calculate the risk of anything any more. I took very few risks before I was ill. But sitting at home playing it safe didn't eliminate risk – I still got ill – so I thought, Why not take a few more risks and have fun while I'm at it? Risk is a deep, dark part of everything, in the cells of all living and dying things. It's unavoidable. I feel it permanently, and I find I am welcoming more of it into my life, seeking it out and playing with it. If I've chosen the risk, I tell myself, it's more under my control. Bo's mumbled 'Fearless' comment was right: I feel like nothing can touch me; I'm beginning to lose sight of fear altogether.

*

In all my reading about free flight, I'm constantly coming across the story of Icarus and Daedalus. Icarus is the most famous flying character of ancient myth. His story is seen as embodying ideas of hubris and wanton risk-taking, of getting carried away and unwittingly challenging nature. But, on returning to the story as it appears in Ovid's

Metamorphoses, I find, to my surprise, not simply a warning against taking too much risk, but a story about the absolute necessity of taking it, in order to be free.

The main character in the story of Icarus is arguably his father, Daedalus, the Athenian engineering genius who designs the famous Cretan labyrinth for King Minos. Daedalus is imprisoned by King Minos, but plans an escape by building wings:

> Then to new arts his cunning thought applies,
> And to improve the work of Nature tries.

Daedalus builds two sets of wings from feathers and wax, one for himself and one for his son, Icarus. He says:

> 'My boy, take care
> To wing your course through the middle air:
> If low, the surges wet your flagging plumes;
> If high, the sun the melting wax consumes:
> Steer between both: nor to the northern skies,
> Nor South Orion, turn your giddy eyes;
> But follow me. Let me before you lay
> Rules for the flight, and mark the pathless way.'

I am pleased that Daedalus's first instruction to Icarus is to not fly too *low* because his wings will become waterlogged by the sea. The story contains warnings against pressing beyond one's limits and the dangers of the upper reaches of one's ambition, but it also warns against the dangers of flying too low, of being too unambitious, of sailing too close to dark, unforgiving waters.

They set off and, of course, Icarus disobeys his father:

> Grown wild, and wanton, more emboldened flies
> Far from his guide, and soars among the skies.

Carried away with the wonder of flying, Icarus flies high, towards the sun, the heat melts the wax and 'Down to the sea he tumbled from on high' and 'found his fate'.

Icarus drowns, but Daedalus flies on successfully to Sicily. He is the arch mythological successful human flyer. The story of Daedalus and Icarus may be a warning of the dangers both of altitude and oceanic depths, but it is also a story of human-engineered flight as a source of power and liberation.

And there's something so exciting about the flights of both Icarus and Daedalus. 'The fate of Icarus frightened no one,' wrote the nineteenth-century French poet Théophile Gautier. 'Wings! Wings! Wings! they cried from all sides, even if we should fall into the sea. To fall from the sky, one must climb there, even for but a moment, and that is more beautiful than to spend one's whole life crawling on the earth.'

*

The summer is easing into autumn, the wind is picking up and Bo has been encouraging me to practise more and more complicated techniques, including more spins and stalls, and crosswind landings. Instead of coming in to land on the strip pointing into the wind, we choose the landing strip at an angle to the wind and I come in with the nose pointing across the strip and into wind, the glider crabbing towards our landing. Bo shows me how to kick the rudder pedal at the last moment so we touch down in a straight line.

One day, in September, Don Gosden, a club pilot and aerobatics instructor, asks me if I'd like to experience an aerobatics flight. Don is a retired Scottish master captain, who spent many years at sea. A mischievous child, he was always in trouble and he still has a defiant streak in him. He took up powered flying in the 1960s and gliding in the 1980s. Aerobatics isn't just thrilling, he tells me, it 'improves your judgement and handling skills . . . helping you understand what the glider and your body can take' during the shifts from plus G-force to negative, and vice versa. A 'red out', he explains, is when minus G-force sends blood rushing to your brain; a 'blackout' is caused by plus G-forces sending your blood rushing away from your head. 'Even if you do blackout in a glider,' he adds, 'provided you've got sufficient height, you'll probably come around again and regain consciousness quickly.'

We haul the heavy glass-fibre K21 glider out of the hangar. It is the first time I've flown in something other than the K13. This is a far more modern machine. We set off into strong ridge lift and fly fast along to Hay Bluff, then back again, flying slightly below the peak. I look out and it seems as if one wing tip is almost touching the hill.

Don keeps us very close to the ridge. I look down and see the purple hue of the heather and the speckled brown shape of a buzzard soaring in circles below us. We push on fast, sheep fleeing up the side of the hill on seeing us; a lamb looks up and I swear I catch its eye. We race along, then head out, away from the ridge, into a thermal to get some lift and some altitude before Don begins the manoeuvres.

We climb to over 4,000 feet, Don does his flight checks, rocks the wings from side to side to mark the beginning of the sequence, and then the fun begins. We speed up to 110 knots, Don gently pulls the stick back, I hear him pressing the rudder pedals in a variety of orders, and we fly upwards at forty-five degrees. We pause for a moment, seeming to hang in the air and I fear we may stall, but then Don makes a turn and we descend and quickly turn again so that we're now pointing in the opposite direction. I'm switched around. We rise up fast, the sky fills my view, then the horizon reappears and all I can see is green fields as we dive downwards, towards the ground, finally pulling out of the manoeuvre to one side.

Gravity shifts and moves inside and around me as Don pulls manoeuvres that take us from plus 4G to negative 1G and back again. I feel the weight of my body increasing and decreasing, almost out of my mouth; the weight of my head feels impossible and I can't move it as I'm pressed awkwardly back into the headrest, my neck slightly twisted. The ground appears in front of me, to one side, then we're heading straight down towards it, then it rocks and rolls to the other side. It's like being inside a turning kaleidoscope.

We move through a series of manoeuvres: a chandelle,

a quarter clover, and a half Cuban. They sound like dances. Then Don takes us into what's called a 'bunt'. He speeds up by dropping the nose and then pulls the nose back up as we continue to speed forward. This gives us a few seconds of negative G. My body is released from gravity and lifts off my seat as bits of grass and rubbish from the floor of the glider rise up too. I'm suspended for one brief, strange moment; it feels like someone paused a movie. Then the movie starts again, gravity reappears and I'm pressed back into my seat. We're both laughing. Don levels us out and tells me to come on to the controls with him. He pushes the stick forward from the back; we speed up. He tells me to pull the stick back gently; the nose rises. I grip the stick as we rise and rise and turn upside down, carving out a great vertical circle in the sky.

Chapter Eight

Into the Wave

I've seen three seasons from the sky, now. The winding, deep lanes that I drive to get to the gliding club have gone through a hot spring, hedgerows crowded with wild flowers, a lush, muddy summer and the winds of autumn, stripping the hedges of their leaves. The music I listen to on the route has shifted over the seasons too, from Bowie to soul to Beethoven to Prince and Swedish folk music. I understand not only how different the landscape looks from the air, as the year passes, but that the sky too is different during each season. In spring, the sky is full of low bulbous cumulus clouds that bring the April showers; in the summer, the cumulus are much higher, fluffier and whiter, and often fade away without dropping any water; in autumn, the sky is more complex, full of layered, lenticular clouds, stacked up like pancakes next to thick, low cumulus. Now it's October, and the sun is low, even at noon. Long, crisp shadows, which never appeared in summer, slice across the landscape.

It's a cold, clear, dark-blue autumn day, with a few cumulus floating about. The airfield is covered in flying spiders' webs, long lengths of silk thread that form sails and allow the tiny spiders to travel huge distances on the wind. A silver shining web, picked out by the low sun, sails slowly past me as I walk to the launch point; I catch it with my forefinger and watch how it trails off into the distance. The sky over the airfield is quiet and empty. The swallows have fledged from their nursery in the hangar and left for Africa.

As Bo and I get ready to launch, the sun shines directly into our eyes. It'll be cold up there, and I'm wearing a woolly hat, thick jumper and hiking jacket.

We take off and I do the aerotow well, holding our position behind the towplane; it feels easy, now. I look down and see the long, narrow shadow of what must be a tall tree, invisible above 1,500 feet, pointing south-east, like the shadow on a sundial.

I release from the tow rope and we head up to the level of the cumulus clouds. Flying along the edge of one, my movements smoother on the controls by now, I look out to the right and see a perfect rainbow-coloured circle with the shadow of our glider moving inside it. It's a 'pilot's glory', Bo tells me, a version of the 'brocken spectre' – a shadow projected on to mist or fog by low sun directly behind an object. A small, clear black silhouette of our glider arcs and banks inside the white centre of a perfect circular rainbow, like a child's badge, the colours glowing, almost seeming to throb. It's an otherworldly sight; hard to believe I'm seeing it at all.

Soon, Bo takes over because he says he can feel something: a smooth lift that's unlike the lumpiness of thermals.

He is recognizing the signs of wave lift, a phenomenon that often happens here in autumn.

Wave was first discovered by German pilots in the 1930s, when they noticed smooth lenticular (lens-shaped) clouds forming behind hills. Flying close to them, they soon discovered powerful invisible wave systems, rippling in layers, far up into the sky, which could take a glider to previously unknown heights. Below these smooth waves was unexpectedly strong broiling turbulence, known as 'rotor'. The phenomenon was further explored, after the Second World War, in the Sierra Nevada, in California. The Sierra Wave Project of the 1950s was a 'mountain meteorology experiment', in which several highly experienced pilots flew gliders high in the wave to take measurements and make observations. The project helped improve our understanding of how the air moves around mountains, and why, in particular, mountains produce tremendous rotor turbulence beneath the rising waves of smooth air. Military and civil aeroplanes were crashing in mountains due to this powerful turbulence and the findings of the Sierra Wave Project helped develop ways to avoid it.

Wave happens more often in the Brecon Beacons and Black Mountains in autumn because the strong seasonal winds bounce up behind the lee side of hills. Bo has found that invisible wave now, and it is taking us slowly and smoothly higher. We pass the altitude at which buzzards and kites soar, and look down on a couple of raptors, which appear as circling black specks in the distance. We head over towards the Brecon Beacons, rising all the time in the continuous, strangely smooth lift. Bo is quiet and concentrating. He's feeling the air to stay in the lift, which is weak but consistent. My instruments are uncovered and my altimeter says we are rising at a speed of three knots. We continue to rise and move through the layer of cumulus clouds to 6,000, then 7,000, then 8,000 feet. I've never been this high in a glider. I look down as the sun catches the curling silver River Usk worming through the valleys below.

We're well above the cumulus clouds, now, and heading into the cloudless Prussian blue. I gape down at the tops of the clouds we normally fly beneath. They're ragged at the edges, curling over themselves at the tops, as though they've been torn to shreds; this is the rotor turbulence below the wave we're rising on, and I can see through the wispier clouds to the landscape below.

And then we reach 10,000 feet, almost two miles up. The curvature of the Earth is just discernible in the bend of the horizon, and I can see the whole body of the Brecon Beacons, all at once, for the first time. What, in my mind, are large hills that dominate the surrounding landscape have become small and compact, dark ripples across the terrain. They are shrouded in a light-blue haze that the stony peaks of Pen y Fan and Corn Du peer up through. Sharp-edged shadows run down one half of a mountain, while the other half is picked out in golden light, turning it a bright emerald green. A valley, lower down, cups a lake of black shadow. The Beacons look like they're covered in a soft, glowing skin, wrinkled in places, like an armpit or a crotch or the creases around a smiling eye.

On the far horizon, the blue sky meets a flat plain of golden orange, below, and it takes me a few moments to realize in astonishment that I'm seeing the west coast of Wales: it's the sea glowing liquid copper. I can see further than I ever have before. The sun is a ball of fire, set low in the sky, glinting off our wings as we circle. We fly in the smooth lift, banking and winding in what feels like slow motion. And time slows down, too, as my attention focuses and I try to take in as much as I can. There's absolutely nothing I can see holding us up, and this, combined with the smoothness of the flight, unlike the bumps and jolts of the thermals, makes it feel even more magical.

Bo circles over the Beacons and then turns back towards the Black Mountains. We fly directly above the valley where I live and I can see that the farmhouse is already in shadow. It's never looked so small to me. I sometimes call home on my mobile when I'm flying above the farm, so Mum and Dad can look up from the yard and see me soaring overhead. But there's no signal up at this altitude. The low sun picks out the russet colour of the dying bracken on the hill above the house, and it glows auburn. We bank and circle directly above the farm; I'm tipped to one side, looking straight down at the grey spot of our yard.

It's getting late, so we head back to the airfield, spiralling down from on high and landing as the sun is beginning to set. As we skim to the end of the airfield and open the canopy, the wind is blowing hard and the oak tree thrashes outside the clubhouse. That was my last flight of the season.

*

The prospect of a winter of no flying horrifies me. I've spent fifty-three hours in the sky, now, and I don't want to come back to earth. The thought of spending a cold, damp winter on the ground in Wales is unbearable; it makes me feel claustrophobic, panicky. I know I am on to something and that flying is part of my ongoing recovery.

A few days later, I talk to Bo about my fears about the winter and my need to keep flying. He can see the impact it is having on me. Bo returns to the southern hemisphere every autumn to teach mountain gliding in the Southern Alps of New Zealand. The mountain soaring school is run by Gavin Wills, and Bo suggests I contact him and tell him about my newfound enthusiasm for gliding.

I email Gavin, outline in brief my recent experiences of life-threatening illness, without naming it, and explain how learning to fly is helping me recover. I ask if it might be possible to come and fly with his school, be a writer in residence perhaps. Gavin gets straight back to me and, with a New World can-do attitude, he says yes, sure, come over. My timing is good. He offers me a room in his old house, which he is just moving out of.

But beneath my excitement, I am worried about something I've kept hidden from Gavin, that Bo had tried to keep hidden from me.

Months ago, Bo lent me a DVD of a flying documentary called *Windborn*. Made in the 1990s, it shows Gavin teaching his teenaged daughter, Lucy, how to fly. The film charts their journey 'in the invisible realm of the wind', and shows a protective father sharing his passion for flying with his daughter, giving her wings. Throughout the story of her training, their relationship is tested as they communicate as only fathers and daughters do.

'You're not using the rudders,' says Gavin.

'I am using the rudders,' Lucy barks back.

After I watched the DVD, I asked Bo about Lucy, wondering if she still flew. He looked down and reluctantly told me that she died about seven years ago. He quickly changed the subject. I wondered about this, and then I twigged. Later, I caught Bo off guard and asked him outright how Lucy died.

'Mmm, breast cancer, I think, possibly, yes,' he said, under his breath.

Lucy died of the illness in her late twenties, after many years of treatment, and I was now the age she would've been. I recalled the warmth of the relationship between Gavin and Lucy in *Windborn* and thought in horror of what they must have been through together.

Now, I am worried about upsetting Gavin by bringing up the illness, and don't feel able to mention it over email because it would seem presumptuous. I figure I just won't tell him; I'll remain vague. But I have to go to New Zealand to fly; something feels intuitively right about it. I've no idea what I'll find there, or what it will mean to fly in a huge mountain range at the edge of the South Pacific, but I know that my psychological recovery depends on it.

There is much to plan, tickets to book and insurance to find (not easy, with my medical history). But I've one more ordeal to face before I can go. A few weeks before my flight to New Zealand, I have a scan. Mum and I sit in the familiar oncology-wing waiting room of the hospital, flicking through magazines. This is truly terrifying, sitting here, helpless once again, staring at photographs of fashion models while surrounded by other cancer patients, people coming and going for blood tests and chemotherapy, women wearing colourful scarves wrapped around their heads; I just want to run screaming from the room, out into the woods next to the hospital.

My name is called, I am prodded and poked, and my chest tapped and listened to. The scan is clear, we are told, and Mum exhales loudly, as though she's been holding her breath for hours.

*

I am free to go. I say goodbye to the swallow-chasing dog, settling down for the winter now the swallows have gone. He sighs by the fire. He has been with me throughout the treatment and was the first 'person', other than my mum, to see my body after surgery. I had called him upstairs (where he's not usually allowed) and into the bathroom as I ran my first bath after the operation. I asked him to sit next to the bathtub so I wouldn't have to face my scarred body on my own.

Mum and Dad drive me to Heathrow and we mill about in a cafe after I've checked my luggage. Then it is time to go. They walk with me to security. Mum looks a bit anxious. They've nursed me through life-threatening illness and now they are trying to smile as they send me off to the other side of the world to fly in dangerous mountains without an engine, with a group of unknown extreme free-flight pilots. I ask so much of them. But I know they are also excited and proud. It's odd how different emotions can crash and travel alongside each other.

As I hug them goodbye, Dad presses something into my hand. I look down and see an enamel brooch of the Welsh and New Zealand flags, joined at the centre.

Part Two

The Southern Alps,
New Zealand

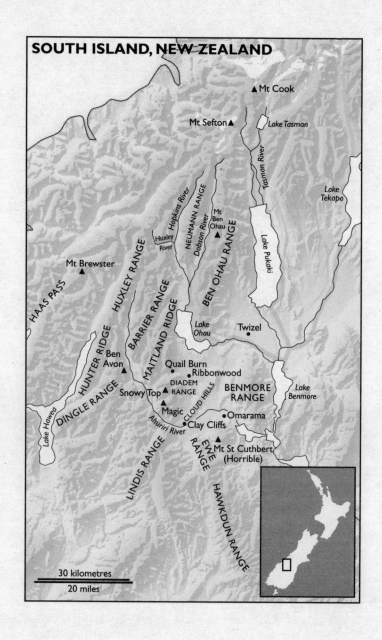

SOUTH ISLAND, NEW ZEALAND

▲ Mt Cook

Mt Sefton ▲

Lake Tasman

Tasman River

Lake Tekapo

Hopkins River

NEUMANN RANGE

Dobson River

Mt Ben Ohau ▲

Huxley River

HUXLEY RANGE

BARRIER RANGE

MAITLAND RIDGE

BEN OHAU RANGE

Lake Pukaki

▲ Mt Brewster

HAAS PASS

HUNTER RIDGE

Ben Avon ▲

Snowy Top ▲

Lake Ohau

Twizel ●

Quail Burn ●

● Ribbonwood

DIADEM RANGE

BENMORE RANGE

Lake Benmore

Magic ▲

CLOUD HILLS

Clay Cliffs ●

● Omarama

DINGLE RANGE

Lake Hawea

Ahuriri River

LINDIS RANGE

EWE RANGE

▲ Mt St Cuthbert (Horrible)

HAWKDUN RANGE

30 kilometres

20 miles

Chapter Nine

Land of the Birds

I'm in the front seat of a high-performance Duo Discus, a sleek glass-fibre two-seat glider with a twenty-metre wingspan. It's at the other end of the performance spectrum from the old wood-and-cloth K13 I fly back in Wales. Where the K13 is shaped like a birch-bark canoe with the broad, solid wings of an eagle, the Duo Discus is a shark with giant albatross-shaped wings: longer, narrower, finer than the K13's. This machine is modern and highly aerodynamic, with a natural elegance to its gorgeously organic shape. It is a piece of sophisticated bio-mimicry.

This glider feels totally different to the K13, too. I am used to sitting up, bent at the hips into an L-shape, with my legs out in front, but in the Duo Discus I'm lying almost supine, the canopy close overhead. It's designed and built by a German company called Schempp-Hirth, co-founded by Wolf Hirth, the pioneer one-legged German glider pilot of the 1930s.

I'm holding on tight to the stick, flying the longest aerotow I've ever flown. By 3,000 feet, my right arm is aching, and I grab the stick with both hands to halve the workload. The only familiar thing here is the voice coming from the back: 'Don't take your eyes off the towplane,' says Bo.

The Duo Discus is far quieter than the K13, which has those noisy cockpit drafts, so Bo speaks relatively softly. The air still howls all around us, but it's distinctly outside the cockpit now and has the deep but distant rumble of an approaching storm. I'm concentrating so hard on the towplane and on hanging on to the stick as we speed along at eighty knots that I don't look about me. Then Bo takes over, releases us from the umbilical cord of the tow rope and circles over what local glider pilots call the Nursery Ridge – a relatively low body of hills, close to the airfield. Finally, I can look properly at the place I've come to fly.

It's December, early summer in the southern hemisphere, and I've been in New Zealand just over a week. We're flying over the airfield that we've just launched from and where I'll be based for the next four months. It is on the edge of a small rural town called Omarama, which is, in turn, on the edge of the MacKenzie Basin, a high, flat plain in the middle of the South Island.

I look around as we circle steeply in tight thermals, and peer up at the smooth, sleek, bright white wing that points into the deep cerulean blue, then turn my head and look down at the other wing and the pale scree-covered mountains below it. The sky is changing quickly, thickening with tall, bulbous cumulus clouds; the ground is dappled and mottled with their shadows, which slip so fast across the landscape that it appears to ripple.

As we rise to 6,000 feet, still well below the cloud base

of the cumulus, I'm looking out at this extraordinary land-scape and sky and waiting to feel something. But I'm numb. I don't know if the jet lag is still having an effect, but nothing is moving in me.

Bo continues to talk from the back: 'The wilder the landscape, the better for me,' he says. 'It's total wilderness, here, in some parts of the South Island.'

But his voice is becoming faint to my ears; I am looking inward and finding a strange blankness there. I've come here, to one of the world's most extreme gliding land-scapes, because I want to know what it is possible to do in an engineless aeroplane – what it is possible for me to do. I've travelled to the other side of the globe to be *here*, doing *this*, and I am unmoved. It's incredible. Bo cannot see my face and must think I'm silent because I'm listening intently to his guided tour of the sky, but in reality tears of frustration are beginning to roll down my stiff cheeks. They take me aback; I am crying for my numb self, the self that has been shocked into silence by the horror of the last few years. Has some part of me shut down? I've been warned that flying here is a big experience and can be scary at first, but I am not afraid and my lack of fear seems to have closed off other feelings as well. There's no euphoria. I am taking no delight in the sky, the place I've come to think of as mine.

The tears continue to fall for about twenty minutes; I make no noise, don't heave, just sit in the front of the cockpit, staring out at the monstrous cumulus clouds passing over the land.

I come back to the flight when Bo tells me to take hold of the stick and fly straight and level over to the mountain ahead of us: Mount Benmore. I look down at the airfield, which is huge – a mile of flat grass, with three giant hangars at its edge.

I fly level at sixty knots, pass over the airfield, 6,000 feet below, and head over a ripple of mountains Bo tells me are the Cloud Hills. They look soft and pillowy, but in fact they're 2,600 feet high, almost the height of Pen y Fan. Here, in this giant landscape, they're low hills, dwarfed by the mountains that surround them. We reach Benmore, and Bo takes over as we begin climbing in the thermals, the rising air lifting up and off the dusty back of the mountain. When I take the controls again, I can feel the strong, muscular mountain thermals as our wing tip catches the edge of one and is forced decisively upwards.

'Turn, turn,' says Bo.

I move the stick, push my foot on the rudder and we bank steeply and circle tightly, the audio vario beeping faster and higher, and at last my heart follows. I am thrilled, desperately grateful to feel again that buzz of ascending on the wind.

The flat, dry plain of the Mackenzie Basin spreads out beneath us, surrounded by mountains at heights of between 3,000 and 7,000 feet. They're brown and grey, with dark patches of stony scree. The plain holds four big turquoise-blue glacial lakes. In the distance, I can just make out Lake Ohau, and the intertwined strands of the Ahuriri River threading along a flat valley bottom. The

Ahuriri is a braided alpine river, which well describes it; it looks like multiple ribbons of woven stone and water.

The mountains, smooth and rounded below me, all look the same at first. Circling and looking down, the view doesn't appear to change as I turn 360 degrees, but, occasionally, light pierces through the cloud layer to spotlight the side of a mountain or a bend in the dark-blue river. The sunshine turns the mountain tops to velvet. The one road that cuts through the plain is a straight grey slash.

This is a totally foreign landscape to me, and I've entered it from above. It's strange to meet it from the perspective of the sky; my first impressions are of patterns and shapes and connections far beyond the human scale. The flying is foreign too, and I'm getting confused by the movement of the sun, which, here in the southern hemisphere, swings around to the north. It is early afternoon and the sun is no longer overhead, but I can't work out the compass direction from it. I'll have to learn to read nature again and flip my memories of its movements on their head. Perhaps it's this sense of being lost that has finally broken open the numbness in me. I'm finding feelings again through being disorientated, shaken up.

As we descend, the Cloud Hills grow large. We soar over the twisting braided river and I fly some of the long wide circuit before Bo takes over and gets on the radio to announce our intention to come in to land: 'Omarama traffic,' he says, 'glider Romeo Zulu downwind left hand zero nine.'

I climb out of the glider with a sense of the vast scales at work here. The cosy patchwork, soft hills and gentle thermals of Wales are far away. This flying is altogether bigger.

A week ago, Gavin Wills and his wife Mandy welcomed me into their home. They had been busy packing up before I arrived, and have now moved into a house they've built next door. I have the whole place to myself, and, after my long journey, I relished the chance to settle into the house and my room, to find some space of my own in this new landscape.

On the wall outside my bedroom is a large framed black-and-white photograph of Lucy, Gavin's daughter from his first marriage. Lucy is naked, leaping into the air, all courage and euphoria in the face of the crisis of her illness. The picture stopped me in my tracks when I first saw it, and I knew straight away that I wouldn't be able to look closely at it for some time. I was standing where Lucy should have been. The evening after my arrival, Gavin and I went for a beer and he told me that the picture was a professional photograph taken the day before Lucy had her mastectomy. Her right breast is blurred in the picture, as though it had already begun to disappear.

Gavin is well over six feet tall, with a big beard and a strong, warm, weather-worn face. He has spent his life exploring the mountains of New Zealand's South Island, first as a geologist, mountaineer and mountain guide, summiting Mount Cook, New Zealand's highest peak, on numerous occasions, and now as a 'sky guide', running the Glide Omarama flying club and taking pilots into the skies above the mountains he knows so well.

He's a kind man, generous with his passion, and, during that evening drink, we talked and talked. For many years, Gavin worked managing avalanches in the Southern Alps, flying his Piper Cub and lobbing explosives out of the window to set off 'controlled' avalanches. He's spent his whole life with his nose pressed right up against the power of these mountains, on the edge of their potential destructiveness. And yet there's a personal, almost physical love for the landscape too. This place is deeply ingrained in Gavin's sense of himself; he is a living, craggy outcrop of these mountains. As he rolled his beer bottle in his hands, Gavin told me how, in 1991, the top of Mount Cook fell off in a giant rock-and-ice landslide, changing its profile forever. He touched his face as he said, 'It was like someone had cut my nose off.'

Gavin has a reputation as a highly experienced, enormously talented pilot, and one who goes to places in his flying where few are skilled enough to follow. He knows what he's doing and wants to stay safe, but he also pushes to the edge. He told me, 'I enjoy exploring the outer limits of my envelope because that's how I learn more about how the atmosphere works and hone my skills.' But, that night, Gavin admitted that, in mountaineering and flying, he enjoys taking risks. His character is a fascinating mixture of the need for absolute control and a willingness to let go, to give in to the power of nature, to experiment.

But then, I suppose he has to. Gavin's sort of flying is relatively new. 'We've been running around on the ground for about two million years,' he said. 'We've been paddling and sailing on the oceans for 10,000 years, but we've been in the air for only about a hundred. The human consciousness about flying is quite limited.'

Gliding has been happening here for sixty of those one hundred years and Gavin's family has been exploring the outer edge of soaring flight since the sport began in the 1930s – it has been part of his world for his entire life. In coming to a landscape so vast and strange to me, it's easy to forget that this is home for Gavin and his family. The skies, lakes and mountains here, their beauty and their drama and their danger, have been and continue to be explored and loved. The cupboards of my bedroom are lined with mountaineering sleeping bags.

*

The day after my first flight, I join the weekly Monday-morning briefing given by Gavin in the 'terminal building'. The Omarama airfield is half a mile from the house where I am staying and the terminal building is a large former aircraft hangar on the edge of the airfield, now broken into meeting rooms and Gavin's offices. On either side of it, long hangars stable Gavin's fleet of high-performance gliders, as well as private pilots' gliders, towplanes, local club gliders and anything else a hangar owner wants to store. Gavin employs a dedicated ground crew to do the work of preparing gliders and stowing them away, so his clients climb in and out of his Duo Discus gliders as spoilt as movie stars.

In the middle of the sparsely populated South Island, amid isolated high-country sheep stations and small rural towns, the flying community at Omarama is global. An international crew of experienced gliding instructors from all over the world come to Omarama to work with Gavin during the southern summer, from Britain, Austria, France, Hungary, Japan, Canada, Australia and Sweden, as well as home-grown New Zealand pilots.

At the briefing, I am introduced to the team properly, and then, in front of Gavin, Bo and a group of visiting pilots, I explain that I'm here as a novice to find out more about soaring, that I've become fascinated by it, that I've been seriously ill and learning to fly is helping me in ways I don't yet fully understand. I am mumbling, looking down at the carpet in front of the group of unfamiliar men. I can't say the words 'breast cancer'; they're too difficult here, too difficult in front of Gavin. I'm a writer, I explain, and will be gathering material during my stay for articles, possibly a book.

Relieved to have got that out of the way, I recede into the background as, one by one, the group of visiting pilots introduce themselves. They have all come here to attend Gavin's mountain soaring course, a week-long immersion in extreme flying, in which pilots are taken by experienced instructors into the Southern Alps on what, for many, will be the longest, highest, most dramatic and exciting flights of their lives. The course includes theoretical instruction in morning lectures and hands-on flying, and the pilots who undertake this course are usually experienced; this is not for novices. Omarama is the place to push your skills in epic adventure flying. I am way out of my depth.

Perched on a high stool, his long legs easily reaching the floor, Gavin opens the week's course by explaining why the conditions here are so ideal for mountain soaring. The Omarama airfield is roughly in the middle of the South Island, on the high, flat plain of the Mackenzie Basin, which is on the edge of the Southern Alps, a range of mountains between 6,000 and 12,000 feet, packed with at least 3,000 glaciers, some of which reach down almost to the sea on the west coast.

The unique nature of this mountainscape and its position amidst the roaring forties, notoriously powerful winds that race across the Southern Ocean before colliding with New Zealand, mean it's an ideal site for unpowered flight: this is one of the windiest inhabited places on earth. The westerly and north-westerly prevailing winds of the Southern Ocean hit the cold peaks of the Southern Alps and, forced upwards, create some of the most powerful lee-wave systems in the world. They have taken gliders almost to the top of the biosphere and carried them over 2,500 kilometres in distance.

The evidence of these lee-wave systems has always been visible. The Maori name for New Zealand is 'Aotearoa', meaning 'land of the long white cloud', and the cloud that refers to is the distinctive north-west arch, a huge lenticular lee-wave cloud that forms like a giant wing and signals the presence of powerful wave lift.

Gavin explains how the unique terrain, hot sun and ferocious winds combine to create an atmospheric engine that generates tremendous power. The Southern Alps funnel the strong winds in and out of steep-sided valleys, creating twisting ridge lift. A southerly wind can be turned down a valley and seem to come from the north. Ridge winds bore up and down the sides of craggy mountains unpredictably, and strong up-currents also mean strong down-currents. The sky is powerful here, and dangerous. The rotor can be strong and there are plenty of rugged crags to crash into. Gavin also points out that the clear, clean air means visibility can be 300 kilometres some-times, so mountains can seem much closer than they actually are – dangerous, if you're getting low and heading for a ridge that you think will have altitude-saving lift moving up and over it, only to discover that it is further away than you thought.

Flying among these rocky mountain giants, a pilot can become isolated, caught between the crags and unable to glide home, and yet this glacier-created geography is blessed with plenty of wide, flat-bottomed valleys, ideal for landing out. Moreover, there are many small airstrips and little landing fields on high-country farm stations, where crop-spraying planes take off and land. This means that, if a glider does land out on one of these remote air-strips, many of them inaccessible by road, a towplane can fly in, once the location of the glider has been radioed, and tow the glider back up or back home.

The unique landscape and its fantastically unstable atmosphere create ideal flying conditions for thermal, ridge, wave and convergence flying (lift where two air masses meet), and you can often experience all four kinds of lift in one day; the conditions can combine and co-operate, or clash together, sometimes creating complex, choppy skies.

Powerful thermals form on many days, with a high cloud base of 7,000, 8,000, even 10,000 feet plus. The mountain thermals here are often 'narrow, feisty, wild little beasts,' says Gavin, 'in which the glider has to be turned sharply, steeply and usually very quickly.'

I look out from the upstairs meeting-room windows at the enormous cumulus clouds rapidly forming above the Benmores. Flying, here, is a test of anyone's handling skills. This is a volatile environment.

*

Whilst I am here, the different instructors at Omarama will squeeze in flying lessons with me between their flights with other visiting pilots. Immediately after Gavin's briefing, Bo has a free couple of hours, so we walk down to the airfield together for my second flight into the New Zealand air.

Today, I decide to cover up my instruments, as I do in Wales. They are new, fancy and beguiling, and I don't want to be distracted by them; I want to get out into the sky.

We take a black T-shirt to the launch point and use it to dress the instrument cover. The cotton drapes over the buttons and knobs, the whole thing looking like a magic trick about to be revealed.

Bo and I take off, I manage most of the aerotow and we climb to cloud base at 6,000 feet, and then practise riding the thermals over the Cloud Hills, looking over to Lake Ohau.

The twisting river slips past my view as I bank steeply. We gain height and fly over towards the small town of Twizel, the audio vario swinging, in seconds, from a high-pitched, fast-beeping squeal to a low growl, responding to the lift and sink of this broiling air. The sky is deep blue and filled with high cirrus clouds above the cumulus scudding over the mountain tops, darkening the ground below. As I look over towards Lake Pukaki, the smell of oranges bursts into the cabin before Bo reaches forward to pass me a few segments. I realize it's a scent I've come to associate with the sky – a glimmer of comfort and familiarity in this strange new landscape.

The New Zealand poet Brian Turner, who lives nearby in Central Otago, writes about the Southern Alps in his poem 'Deserts, for instance':

> The loveliest places of all
> are those that look as if
> there's nothing there
> to those still learning to look.

I think he meant that the South Island landscape looks

empty at first, until you start to see its details. I am learning to look at the sky, to adjust to the wildly swinging audio vario and the powerful, tight thermals, but I'm having to learn to look at this new landscape too.

In coming to the other side of the world, I've broken the cycle of the seasons, leapfrogging winter to arrive in late spring. And I don't recognize the signs of seasonal change here. Back in Wales, I notice the smallest shifts in the turning year: the first snowdrops, first hedgerow celandines, wood anemones, when the blackbirds start to get restless and crows fly past with sticks in their beaks. Here, I don't know what to look for and I misread the landscape, at first. Noticing patches of bare rock and jumbled stone, I immediately think, Oh, there's some kind of ancient ruin, an abandoned human settlement. I have a European aerial archaeological eye that expects to see evidence of human habitation everywhere, remnants of ancient sites rearing up out of the ground, revealing the past that's buried deep in the soil, layer upon layer, as it is in Wales. But then I remember that, no, there have hardly been humans here at all. The Maoris arrived some 800 years ago, the Europeans even more recently, and only a few will have travelled into this remote and inhospitable landscape.

And beyond this is the wider knowledge that New Zealand has very few native mammal inhabitants at all. This is the land of the birds. In fact, the only mammals indigenous to New Zealand are three kinds of bat, seals on the coast and the whales in New Zealand's waters. The islands that make up New Zealand broke away from the larger continent,

Gondwanaland, eighty million years ago. Unreachable except by air, they were, until the Maoris' arrival, islands of birds – some of the most extraordinary ever to have evolved.

The coast of New Zealand is home to the most diverse collection of seabirds in the world, and some of the most remarkable, including the sooty shearwater, which flies a 64,000-kilometre round trip each year, the longest animal migration ever recorded, and the wandering albatross, the largest flying bird now in existence and the greatest soaring bird in the world.

Because the only indigenous mammals to live in the interior of the two islands of New Zealand could fly, many of the country's unique birds evolved to become ground-dwellers, losing their power of flight. New Zealand is home to the world's largest population of flightless birds – their remnant wings stumps, their feathers almost returned to fur. About 800 years ago, New Zealand was a final outpost of purely avian life, where birds were free to waddle along the forest floor, scratching around for food and carving out spaces on the ground for eggs and young, unthreatened by ground-dwelling predators.

But returning to the ground, of course, left these birds extremely vulnerable in the rapid ecological transformation brought about by the arrival of humans, and many of New Zealand's flightless birds are now extinct. The most famous of these is the large moa, which could grow to be twelve feet tall and spent millions of years as the archipelago's largest animal. The moa knew only one predator before humans: the equally enormous Haast's eagle. This giant eagle once lived on the South Island and is the largest eagle ever known to have existed, with a four-metre wingspan. It preyed on moas, and both grew large through a process known as 'island gigantism', where limited predators and an abundance of food mean animals grow increasingly big. The Haast's eagle became extinct around 1400, when the moa disappeared, hunted to extinction by the Maoris.

A later casualty was the whekau or laughing owl, which was endemic to New Zealand and plentiful in the nineteenth century. Named for its hysterical shriek, it had, over many generations, become a ground feeder, chasing prey on foot. It could still just about get airborne, but had lost the skilful silent flight of its fellow owls. The introduction of stoats, cats and weasels by European settlers proved too much for the laughing owl, and it had become extinct by 1914.

Today, New Zealand's flightless birds include several kinds of kiwi, six different types of penguin, the brown flightless rail, called a weka, the colourful blue takahe and the bizarre kakapo, a green parrot that sits in a dusty bowl and booms out into the night, sending reverberations across the ground to entice a female. There are even flightless ducks in New Zealand: the Auckland Island teal and the Campbell Island teal. Other birds are on their way to evolved flightlessness and have become poor fliers, such as the kokako, the saddleback, the rifleman and the rock wren, a fat little bird that hops from place to place eating grubs and insects.

Even though I know evolution is about filling a niche, I can't help but find the process of evolved flightlessness troubling. The movement from the ground into the sky feels like a linear progression onwards and upwards – that's certainly what it has been for me. As Bo and I soar above Twizel, I find myself hunting for birds, willing them to be in the sky around us, showing us the best path through the thermals. But there aren't any; they are all below us, on the ground, and I find it hard not to see the evolution of flightlessness as a backwards step, even though I know it is a matter of survival. We've gone in opposite directions, these New Zealand birds and me.

It's late December, my third flight here, and Bo and I are flying in strong thermals over Quail Burn Gap towards the Diadems and the Ribbonwood Gap, looking at Lake Hawea in the distance. This is the furthest I've travelled from the airfield yet. The sun is fierce. I'm wearing my usual blue cloth hat, cheap sunglasses and factor fifty suncream. Circling on the edge of Ribbonwood, I can see the shore of Lake Pukaki and the Mackenzie Basin reaching out towards it.

The larger features of the landscape are becoming familiar, the shapes of the mountains and valleys sharpening and coming into focus. At first, it was like looking at a large crowd of people, whose indistinct faces blur into a single mass. Now, the long, low ripples of the Cloud Hills and the Chain Hills, the yellow gash of the Clay Cliffs, the elegant bend of the Ahuriri River as it passes along the valley bottom, the sway back of the Omarama Saddle, the dark, lumpy, craggy heap that is Saint Cuthbert, right above the airfield, known as Mount Horrible, and the striped, rounded belly of Mount Ben Ohau, jutting out into Lake Ohau, itself a slice of blue sky that's fallen to the ground and lies at the foot of the mountain, are all beginning to take on a distinct shape and character for me.

From the air, I'm beginning to recognize these shapes and the spaces between them, but to understand the landscape better, I need to spend time on the ground. The Omarama terminal building walls are covered with large maps, and so I spend one hot afternoon, when all the instructors are too busy to give me a flying lesson, studying them.

The biggest map shows the Southern Alps stretching down the west of the South Island, and I trace them from north to south with my finger. Many of the names here read like exclamations or emotional expressions: the Remarkables Range, Magic Mountain, Hope River; there are several Mount Miserables, and a Mount Aspiring, Possibility Col, Solution Range, Mount Bitterness, Futurity Rock, Mount Awful, the Valley of Darkness and the Great Unknown.

What's most notable on a cursory look, though, is the mix of Maori and European names. They feel completely different in the mouth. The Maori words are full of hard ks and gs, and soft vowels, such as o, au and ea; the European names are more likely to feature th, st and b. Saying the names out loud – Pukaki, Ohau, Hawea, Wanaka, Wakatipu, Rangiora, Te Anau – feels completely at odds with Saint Cuthbert, Rabbiter's Peak, Mount Martha, the Buscott, Billy Burn, Flood Burn, Saint Bathans, as though the landscape tastes different in each culture.

Some places on the map are given two names: one Maori, the other European. The highest peak in the Southern Alps is Aoraki / Mount Cook, its official name since the 1998 treaty settlements between the Maoris and Pakehas (non-Maori New Zealanders of European descent), in which many dual names for the landscape were established. The mountain range as a whole has two names: the Southern Alps and Ka Tiritiri O Te Moana. Then there's Haast Pass / Tioripatea, Mount Aspiring / Tititea, Franz Josef / Waiau and Fox Glacier/ Te Moeka O Tuawe, to name just a few. Aoraki / Mount Cook is the only site where the Maori name officially comes first.

While the land and its names are all strange to me, this bilingualism has a familiar echo. Living on the border between England and Wales, I'm used to reading signs twice, silently naming places in both Welsh and English: Aberhonddu / Brecon, Y Fenni / Abergavenny, Abertawe / Swansea, Caerdydd / Cardiff. A familiar town or hill that, to me, has a singular nature, has two names, and the place itself seems to fall into the crack between them. The official name of the hills in which I live is the Black Mountains / Y Mynyddoedd Duon. And yet, from the sky, these different names, these man-made definitions and boundaries, don't matter, are totally invisible.

I'm used to exploring a landscape that holds cultural tensions and competing versions of history between its dual names, each one jostling for position to be said first or considered most authentic. I recognize the curious effect this has, where each time you name a place, even inside your own head, you must choose sides. I never know which side to take, uncertain of my position, illegitimate one way or another, not enough of either.

Though born in England, Dad is half Russian, his mother a stateless émigré born to White Russian parents who escaped to China after the Revolution. My Russian grandmother, Galena, is bilingual and I grew up hearing her talk Russian with my great-grandmother, Nina, and my great-aunt, Ludmilla, so I understood early on that the real world exists somewhere in the spaces between languages. I like the dual naming in the border country of Wales because it reminds me that a place and its names are not identical, the landscape will always be at one remove from the language we name it with, our words will always be the finger pointing to the moon rather than the moon itself.

New Zealand might not be strewn with human remains or the imprints of settlements, but the controversies over the history of human relations here is written in the vowels and consonants competing to be spoken. Saying 'Aoraki / Mount Cook' out loud sounds awkward. Most people in the flying community call it 'Mount Cook' and I feel like a pretentious outsider saying 'Aoraki' in front of them. But, of course, it's not some binary edifice with two opposing identities. The only way I'm going to get to know it will be to fly over and around the mountain.

Chapter Ten

The Moon is Upside Down

The first glider to reach New Zealand's South Island in 1950 was an English Slingsby Prefect, and the second was a post-Second World War requisitioned German glider, a 1930s Weihe, given by Gavin's uncle, Philip Wills, to Dick Georgeson and now hanging from the ceiling of the foyer of Queenstown airport, like a child's giant mobile. Dick Georgeson is considered the pioneer of wave soaring, and on the wall of the briefing room at Glide Omarama there's a photo of a nine-year-old Gavin talking to Dick as he sits in a glider. Dick grew up locally, on Irishman's Creek sheep station, watching the kahu hawks flying in the thermals over the tussock grass, and he was the first to fly the wave system here when, in 1950, aged twenty-eight, he soared to 10,000 feet in the Slingsby wood-and-cloth glider, with no oxygen, in a sky that Gavin frequently describes as 'an Antarctic-like environment, but without breathable air.'

The wave is the kind of lift that the Southern Alps are most famous for and it's extremely complex, requiring sophisticated knowledge, experience and understanding to fly it. One day, waiting for the wind to pick up, I ask

Gavin about Dick and he explains that Dick was the first pilot in the world to explore wave flying across the wind, rather than up or down wind. Because the South Island is so narrow, if Dick flew up or down wind in the wave, he would soon head out to sea, so he flew along the prevailing north-westerly wave, and that allowed him to fly the length of New Zealand without heading out to sea. He demonstrated to glider pilots across the world how long-distance wave flying could be done.

The Southern Alps are the mountain range in which New Zealand mountaineer Edmund Hillary cut his teeth, before he reached the summit of Everest in 1953. They're much lower than the Himalayas, but the weather changes quickly. 'It wasn't until I travelled widely overseas', wrote Hillary, 'that I came to appreciate the mountains of New Zealand both for their beauty and for the challenge they presented the enthusiastic climber . . . The weather can be warm and balmy one moment and tumultuous the next – a full scale nor'west storm is more to be feared than any Himalayan blizzard.' As Hillary explored the mountains from the ground, Dick navigated the skies above them. He would go on to fly distances of over 1,000 kilometres and, in 1960, he flew to 34,500 feet, right over the country's signature long white cloud: 'I was right over the top of the nor'west arch and looking down the dazzling cliff face of cloud stretching five kilometres below me', he wrote afterwards.

What I don't realize, until the end of that conversation with Gavin, is that Dick is still at Omarama, living in a chalet at the edge of the airfield. A few days later, I walk over to meet him, giddy with excitement. Now in his nineties, tiny, almost blind, he is full of stories. He describes the wave as a 'wind of meaning' that has given sense to his life. I ask him how he coped when, at 35,000 feet, his air brakes froze and he realized he was suffering from signs of hypoxia when he turned his oxygen *off* rather than up. 'The antidote to fear,' he tells me, 'is fascination.'

Most mornings, after the weather briefing, where the conditions for the day ahead are discussed, I walk over to the Kahu Cafe, on the edge of the airfield – the unofficial clubhouse for the flying community at Omarama. An eclectic range of old, worn, comfy sofas and armchairs sit at odd angles along the wooden veranda outside the one-room cafe building. Wooden barrels overflow with flowers and herbs. A giant metal silhouette of a kahu hawk flies across the outside wall of the cafe. Dagmar is in charge here. Originally from Germany, she, her mother and four sisters were forced to walk from the east to the west of the country to escape the Russians during the war. After fleeing, they survived the rest of the war on the outskirts of Dresden, watching the city being firebombed from the edge of the forest. Dagmar came to New Zealand on an oceanographic research ship in the 1970s and never left. She married a mountaineer, had a child and spent many years managing mountaineering camps, high in the Southern Alps. Her daughter, Mayan, is a world-champion rock-climber. Now in her seventies, Dagmar is quiet, self-contained. Her husband died many years ago. I don't know where she lives, but on hot nights she sleeps out on one of the sofas on the veranda.

Spending time at the Kahu Cafe is a great way to get to know fellow pilots. Dagmar serves excellent coffee and freshly made muffins that everyone here finds hard to resist, and most days the conditions don't usually come right for flying until the early afternoon, so there are long mornings to spend in the Kahu, listening to stories.

Each day, I find myself seeking out a new face, a new list of achievements. I meet Justin Wills, Gavin's cousin and son of Philip Wills, one of the driving forces in establishing the British gliding movement. Justin was born and educated in Britain and has a certain Englishman's reserve, but he cannot help but impress as he tells me about his father. Philip Wills flew in competition with Hanna Reitsch in the 1930s, took part in anti-invasion manoeuvres during the Second World War (Philip was among a group of pilots towed to 10,000 feet over the English Channel to fly as radar target practice in order to test whether the British radar systems would pick up German troop-carrying gliders) and broke numerous world records.

As in Wales, women glider pilots are a minority at Omarama, but this is the home of epic adventure gliding and so the women I do meet are at the top of their game. Two world-record breakers are Jenny Wilkinson and Yvonne Loader.

During my second week in Omarama, Yvonne sits down to talk over a coffee, our conversation punctuated by glances through the window to the windsock on the airfield. Yvonne used to fly in competitions as a power pilot, but later took up gliding.

'Power flying is all on one emotional level,' she tells me, 'but with gliding there's both extreme exhilaration and extreme frustration.'

In 1988, she secured the women's altitude world record in a Nimbus glider, flown from Omarama to Mount Cook, where she climbed to 37,000 feet. She grins as she remembers that flight. 'The world from that height is so beautiful,' she says. 'The mountains become little pimples below you.'

It must have been a thrill for Yvonne to soar so high after the limitations of powered flight. You can go higher in a glider because the engine of a small power plane can't cope in the thin air at high altitudes. And then, of course, there's the feel of it. No engine growling to mask the air around you.

'I love wave flying,' Yvonne says. 'It's like riding on velvet.'

There are also people staying on the edge of the airfield who are part of the community, but no longer fly. A tall Canadian known as 'Pipe' escapes the harsh Canadian winter each year to live on the Omarama airfield in a caravan for six months. He is one of the few people brave enough to drive the hang-gliders, who also come to fly in these mountains, up the extremely steep gravel zigzag track to the top of Magic Mountain, where they launch into the sky. But most days he folds himself into one of the worn-out armchairs on the cafe veranda and smokes his

pipe, exuding a wise calmness that is a welcome antidote
to the manic energy of some pilots after a good flight,
when the air on the veranda seems to crackle. Pipe occasionally offers up a gnomic remark that hangs in the air
along with his pipe smoke.

Every Thursday evening, Gavin, his crew and anyone
who's come to fly with them have dinner at the Kahu. I
join them one warm December night and find myself sitting between Gavin and Mandy. We are eating lamb shanks
in a steaming Moroccan sauce, and about twenty-five
people are crammed around the long table, their backs
pressed up against the cafe walls. Bo is sitting at the other
end of the table, and I grin each time I catch his eye.

Today is an emotional day for Gavin; he's become a
grandfather for the first time – his son, George, from his
first marriage, has just had a little boy. Gavin is effusive,
and as he stands to announce the news to everyone, he
towers over the long dinner table. After we have toasted
the family's new arrival, Gavin begins to talk about his
beloved daughter, Lucy, George's sister. He wonders aloud
what she would have been doing now, had she survived,
and, as he speaks, there is a distinct shift in atmosphere
– many of the people here have known and worked
together for years, most knew Lucy, and the sense of that
loss, of there being someone missing from this celebratory
evening, is powerful.

Gavin's openness, about Lucy and her illness and his
own pain, is amazing to me, and suddenly I know I need
to tell him the truth, I need to reciprocate. Later in the

course of the meal, we talk and I tell him that I too have had breast cancer, that this is the illness from which I'm recovering. It is why I'm here, I say, because flying is helping me come to terms with the changes the illness has wrought in me physically and psychologically. I admit that I wasn't sure whether to mention it, that I know about Lucy, that I don't want to bring back painful memories — that I'm the age she would have been. As he asks informed questions about my diagnosis and treatment, Gavin's expression is purely kind and welcoming, and I am flooded with relief. I think he understands why I have come.

The next day, I walk up to Gavin and Mandy's new house. Gavin makes some tea and we sit on the veranda to talk. The house is positioned below the circuit that gliders usually take when coming in to land, so Gavin has an excellent view of people flying in and can comment on their approach. He must be one of the few people who enjoy living under a flight path. The view looks out across to the Benmores and the Cloud Hills, and down to the Ahuriri River, which edges the garden. Held by this immense vista, our conversation turns quickly to the darkest, most painful thing a person can talk about: the death of their child.

I am afraid to hear this story because I fear it might become my own, but I resist the urge to change the subject. Gavin smiles and tells me stories of Lucy as a plucky little girl, and as a courageous and demanding young woman. He tells me about her bravery as a child, joining in his mountain and flying adventures, and how he thinks she took some of the courage she developed then into her confrontation with illness. Talking about Lucy brings her momentarily back, and Gavin's eyes are shining.

For the first time in months, I start talking about my own experience, about the fear and loneliness of cancer, about the shame of it and the sheer exhausting drudgery of treatment. As I speak, he listens intently, nodding in understanding.

Gavin tells me about the years Lucy and the family had spent trying to find cures, and then how, when they realized her body really couldn't be saved, their focus shifted to spiritual health in the face of the cancer.

'The thing about Lucy,' Gavin says, 'is that she grew so mentally and spiritually powerful in the face of the cancer, that she was the one supporting us in our grief and confusion.'

As Lucy entered into the labour of dying well, with absolute fearlessness, Gavin was forced to watch the terrible suffering of an unstoppable illness, and it transformed him. He was with her when she died, without pain relief, years after the initial diagnosis.

Lucy's illness and death was a profound experience, and it broke him open. There was no escaping the soul-wrenching loss; all he could do was learn to live inside it. Now, the awful suffering has brought him closer to some kind of truth that he's still working through. He tells me that the pain of the loss never goes away; it doesn't diminish. 'You line it with flowers,' he says, 'so you can visit there.' Here is a father who has lost his precious daughter but has found a way to recommit to life without turning away from or denying the pain of his loss. I hope that, in this conversation, we are visiting that painful place and bringing fresh flowers.

By now, it is late afternoon, and we hug on the veranda. Gavin is so tall that I only come up to his chest. It makes me feel like a child again.

On the way back home, I find myself circling around how Lucy's death might have affected Gavin. Perhaps his courage to face challenges in mountains and in powerful skies has developed his capacity to withstand risk, and maybe these strengths helped him face Lucy's illness. He's been familiar with risk throughout his life, growing up in an adventurous flying family determined to push the boundaries. His father, Matthew, almost died in a gliding accident when Gavin was in his early teens, and Gavin has lost many friends in mountaineering and flying accidents; he lives with risk, uncertainty and loss. And yet I also wonder if, when Lucy died, he lost something so precious that he passed through some kind of barrier. The flying he does may be controlled, but only to a point – it's incredibly dangerous. Perhaps he's already got one foot on the other side.

Back, alone, in the lower house, where Lucy once lived, I make something to eat. In the kitchen drawer, I find, seven years after her death, Lucy's herb chest, full of turmeric and other spices. I bring it to my nose and inhale the aromas. I scan the bookshelf next to her photograph, take down a book, open it and see her name handwritten

on the front page: *Lucy Wills*. I run my forefinger over the
ink and shiver. The boundary between this world and the
other has thinned momentarily, is close, here, in this handwritten name in a book, in this photograph of a naked
woman leaping into the air, in the smells of the herbs
and in where I am standing, looking out of the big glass
windows of the kitchen, on to the waving tussock grass.

Later that evening, I walk outside into the garden.
'Omarama' means 'place of moonlight' and tonight the
almost full moon looks odd, its pockmarks and shadows
scrambled. Its glow is familiar, but wrong somehow, and I
realize that, to my northern-hemisphere perspective, it's
upside down. I'm so far away from home that the moon
has flipped over. I stand in the dark with my feet apart and
bend over. Blood rushes to my head, my ears fill with
white noise, but the face of the familiar man in the moon
suddenly appears. I stand up and the moon is on its head
again. I bend over. This is what it's like, I think, trying to
see the world as it was before, even after it has been
turned upside down. It's an effort, blood rushes and pools
in places it shouldn't. Trying to make things familiar when
they are permanently changed involves contortions that
aren't healthy. Gavin's world was turned upside down
with the loss of Lucy and he's learned to live with it that
way; my world, too, has been flipped on its head, but in
some ways I'm still contorting myself to see it as it was
before. I stand up, resolving to face the unfamiliar moon.

*

One hot late-afternoon in mid-December, Gavin, Mandy and I set off for a walk out into the bush, to the Ahuriri River. The dry ground radiates heat upwards, so it's a relief when we reach the bank of the river, glacial blue and flowing fast. Gavin strides confidently out into the water whilst Mandy stands with me at the edge and offers to link arms. We step together into the water, with her on the upside of the flow, taking the brunt of the current. A few steps in, the water up to my thighs, pushing hard against me, I freeze. A conversation with Phil Plane, a flying instructor, over dinner at the Kahu, about the risks of drowning echoes in my head. Drowning is so common here that it's known as 'the New Zealand death'. I fear that, if I lift another foot, I'll be swept downstream.

'I can't do it,' I hear myself say.

Mandy and I are still in the river for a moment and then we cautiously edge backwards to the riverbank. Gavin, now on the other side, starts slowly striding back across towards us. He makes for a biblical figure, out in the middle of the rushing river.

Once on our side, he picks up a long stick, passes it to Mandy and they stand either side of me, telling me to hold on to it with both hands in front. We all grip it. Gavin explains that we will hold the stick at the same angle as the water is flowing and walk diagonally across the river, moving downstream so we're not fighting the current. He tells me not to let my feet off the bottom of the river-bed, but to shuffle them forward, feeling my way around boulders and rocks.

Holding the stick, my shoulders pressed into Gavin on one side and Mandy on the other, we step into the water together. Just before we reach the middle of the river, I look ahead: 'I don't think I can cross all the way,' I say, feeling the first twinge of anxiety for a long time.

We slow and stop momentarily. Gavin and Mandy are silent, and then Gavin says, calmly but forcefully, 'We're almost there, now, so we may as well keep going.'

Gavin and Mandy press on and, between them, I've no choice other than to follow. I feel my feet shuffling along the rocky bottom, a few inches at a time, and then the ground begins to shallow and we rise up out of the water. Stepping from the river on to the bank, water pouring out of my hiking boots, I am both elated to have made it across and embarrassed that I had found it hard. I know that Gavin would not have let us turn back.

We walk upstream to a spot where the river slows and pools. There is no point in getting out of my sodden walking boots, but I strip down to knickers and T-shirt and step again into the river. The water is turquoise and slow moving, and so cold I'm forced to suck in a breath. I swim over towards the opposite bank where willows bend down towards the river and white sun-bleached rocks and wood are scattered along the riverbank. There is no silt and the glassy-clear water magnifies the riverbed, the sun creating scaly crocodile-skin patterns on the rocks below. The dusty, hot, dry mountains of the high country are in the distance, Mount Horrible lumpy and looming.

Mandy and I paddle downstream, where the current

quickens as the route of the river narrows, and I let myself be picked up by the flow and whooshed backwards, out into the main course of the river, where it slows again. Back at the pool, Mandy and I take turns to let go and rush downstream, while Gavin swims in the depths. It is a joy to be held up by the glassy water, rippling all about me, to be immersed in the cool frenzy of it, and being here with Gavin and Mandy feels somehow gentle, right – like our connection has been established.

On the way home, we cross the river again, and again I am held between Gavin and Mandy's strong shoulders, the three of us solid and safe as the water curls around us.

Chapter Eleven

Native Sky

I've left the Mackenzie Basin for the first time and, with sixty kilometres behind us, any psychological rope of connection with the airfield is broken. I've never flown so far from my starting point. It's a hot day, there's a high cloud base, 10,000 feet, and strong winds. I'm flying in ridge lift along the Dingle Range, following the shapes of the rocks, drawing their profile in the air, keeping close to one side of the top of the mountains' spine. The air moving around the rocks is like a warped mirror image of the mountains, rippling and bending, a distorted echo reaching up into the sky and taking us higher and higher.

I circle and climb in the thermal, looking down into the dark rocky crags with gullies picked out in icy white by miniature glaciers. The mountains turn on their sides as I bank steeply.

'It's endlessly intriguing,' says Bo, 'the difference moving just a hundred yards can make. Even on the scale of these mountains, you work on micro-meteorology; small movements make a big difference to the details you see.'

We track over on to the Hunter Ridge, a long spine of

rock like a lizard's back, and ahead I see the dark-blue expanse of Lake Hawea. As we fly along the edge of the long lake, I start to feel trapped and claustrophobic. I wriggle silently in my seat. My brain is registering the sharp peaks below, the expanse of cold blue water and the steep-sided valleys. Bo knows these mountains well and where the land out options are, but, aware that we're several mountain ranges from Omarama, my brain churns over and seems to shrink like a squeezed sponge.

I open the vent on the left side of the canopy and cold air slaps my cheek. I take a swig of water. After a while, my discomfort recedes and I relax, and let the joy of being here well up. I fly along the knobbly ridge and, concentrating on the feel of the air, I clearly discern a kind of sweet spot above and slightly to one side of the spine. I follow it fast, making small adjustments to stay in that spot, my confidence surging as we track along. The mountain flies past beneath me. I've a tail wind and am eating up the ground.

In the distance, I see the dark pointed triangle of Mount Aspiring at more than 9,900 feet, jutting up above the peaks that surround it. I look down to the lake and see the narrow pass between Hawea and Lake Wanaka, and further north to where the Wilkin River twists down a narrow valley. From where we are flying, it is like we are at the centre of a giant octopus, as ridges and valleys reach out in every direction and wind away into the distance.

New Zealand looks so extraordinary from above – an elemental, wild terrain – it's no wonder that it has become the raw material for fantasy landscapes in the movies. New Zealand's film industry is thriving and, whilst I am here, Peter Jackson is in the process of making *The Hobbit*. The raw footage of the land will be digitally manipulated, virtually out of all recognition, but nevertheless the South Island is the visual baseline of Middle Earth; it's also the base for Skull Island (the home of King Kong), Narnia and Pandora, the Edenic planet where James Cameron's avatars explore the alien forest.

But, through snippets of conversations I overhear in the Kahu, I'm coming to understand that, beyond its image as an archetypal landscape of mountains, volcanoes, glaciers, rivers, forests, sandy beaches, waterfalls and lakes ideal for manipulating into imaginary worlds, this land is steeped in controversy and crisis on the ground.

Over a series of regular barbecues at Gavin's house, it becomes apparent that the ongoing arguments over New Zealand's history are a subject of huge importance to the community here. Across New Zealand, relations between Maoris and Pakehas are often strained and most obviously when it comes to disagreements over the legitimacy of the Treaty of Waitangi. Signed in 1840 between 500 Maori chiefs and the British Crown, it was New Zealand's founding document, and attempted to signal a partnership between the British and the Maori people, as well as establishing New Zealand as a British colony. But the treaty has been mired in controversy from the start, some suggesting that there was no real agreed understanding between the British and the Maoris about what the treaty meant in practice, in part due to problems in the translation of the document and the subtle differences between terms such as 'governance' and 'sovereignty' in each language. After over a century of conflict between the Maoris and the British, and campaigning by the Maori people, the Waitangi Tribunal was set up in 1975 to look more deeply into the treaty and its role in the history of Maori–Pakeha relations, particularly in regard to land purchases and ownership. But disagreements about the document and its contemporary implications are ongoing still.

And, behind these human controversies, I begin to realize, are ecological ones. Flying over the Ahuriri on our way back to the airfield, I spot the multicoloured blue, purple, pink and white of a braided riverbed covered in lupins. It's a beautiful sight, but when I point it out to Bo, he replies, 'They're a weed, a pest.' This happens often, in the Kahu, when I remark on the beauty of a tree or a bush, and I'm told that it's an invasive species and shouldn't be here at all. The appreciation of flora and fauna here is shaped by whether it's an introduced species or a native.

I find this most difficult with regard to the wildlife. One afternoon, when there's no flying in the offing, I borrow Bo's car and drive up the gravel track of the Ahuriri Valley to look more closely at the river and its route. As I drive back down the valley, grumbling to myself about a missing earring that must have fallen out when I was standing on the riverbank, I am amazed to see numerous brown hares leaping on their strong back legs along the edge of the road, their black-tipped ears waving this way and that. They're large and sleek, a cross between a kangaroo and a rabbit. A rare sight on the farm in Wales, the hare is a sacred and secretive creature, to me, strangely homeless in the way it sleeps in flattened areas of grass and lives so lightly on the ground. But, when I get back to Omarama and talk excitedly about the hares, their strange gait and mesmerizing ears, I am told that they are pests, along with the rabbits, the plague of which has ruined many high country farms in the past.

In New Zealand, conservation issues take centre stage. Kiwis, I soon see, are passionate about their land, and efforts to save their endangered national symbol are a high priority. It's a matter of national sadness that most New Zealanders will never see a kiwi in the wild, only in nature reserves or zoos, and, in an effort to turn the kiwi's fortunes around, New Zealand's Department of Conservation is attempting to reduce, if not eradicate altogether, the population of pests (including possums, stoats, rabbits, hares, weasels and hedgehogs) that threaten the kiwi and other flightless birds. Their controversial policy (unpopular with many) involves spreading pellets poisoned with 1080, sodium fluoroacetate, across the ground from helicopters.

Conservationists are attempting to undo the work of nineteenth- and early-twentieth-century Europeans who introduced all kinds of birds and mammals into New Zealand, resulting in native species being made extinct or forced to the brink of extinction. Beyond farm animals, the Europeans brought over a veritable Noah's Ark of creatures to release. As T. E. Donne of the Department of Tourist and Health Resorts put it in 1924, 'Nature neglected New Zealand in providing game animals; man has remedied the omissions.'

Around 1850, the first red deer were released. In the 1860s 'acclimatization societies' were formed to coordinate the stocking of the country with foreign birds and mammals. In 1867, starlings, yellowhammers, skylarks, chaffinches, blackbirds and thrushes were introduced from England. Nightingales failed to establish. Fallow deer, Asian chital deer and sika were also introduced, as well as pheasants, quails and partridges, all for hunting. A cage load of red foxes were released, but failed to take hold. These were followed, a few decades later, by a North American bestiary that included Canada and snow geese, various species of duck, moose (which didn't take to their new home), raccoons, terrapins, owls, Himalayan tahr and Virginian deer.

Emperor Franz Josef of the Austro-Hungarian Empire sent a gift of a shipment of chamois to be released into the Southern Alps; they were set free close to Mount Cook and still thrive there.

This introduced menagerie effectively traumatized the native ground birds and plants by eating flora that had never evolved any protection from browsing animals. At least fifty species of bird have become extinct in New Zealand since humans – including the Maoris, who brought with them dogs, rats, cats and pigs – arrived on the islands.

The Department of Conservation is now trying to undo this damage to preserve what's left of the globally unique ecology of New Zealand. It is a grand and terrible task – a mission impossible, some say. But they have made great strides on some of the small islands outlying the mainland, where they have managed to eradicate all pests and create nature reserves for some of the most vulnerable endangered birds and plants.

Every morning at Omarama, walking across the airfield to the Kahu, I hear the melodious liquid yodelling of the Australian magpies (also known as the bell magpie, organ bird or flute bird – their Latin name translates as 'flautist'). They carol together in voices that range across four octaves and ripple through the air with an electric pulsing quality. Large, black and white, they reminded the European colonists in Australia of magpies and they called them so, but they're really a species of butcher-bird. They were introduced from Australia to the South Island in the 1860s and are now categorized as an invasive species.

Sitting on the cafe veranda, I hear blackbirds singing in the bushes; these birds were originally shipped over to New Zealand in the 1860s by colonists homesick for their melodies. When I close my eyes, the blackbirds' song takes me back momentarily and I almost believe I have travelled the 12,000 miles home, but as soon as the exotic fluting of the magpies interjects, I know I am far away. The birdsong in the air about the airfield is my soundtrack on the ground, dominated by the blackbird and the Australian magpie. But both are non-native birds here, widely considered ecologically inauthentic. I listen to their music and try not to let that knowledge ruin their song for me.

Back in the air, as Bo and I continue flying along the Hunter Range, searching for lift, I wonder if the only truly native part of this landscape is the sky above it. This sky is surely just as it was when the Maoris first arrived and noticed the South Island's distinctive long white cloud. Flying inside this native sky is to be momentarily lifted above the intractable problems on the ground. We turn and fly east across the Barrier Range, out into the Mackenzie Basin and then the fifty kilometres back to Omarama.

The most recent crisis of the South Island's extraordinary landscape came in February 2011, when the Canterbury region was struck by a 6.3-magnitude earthquake. Its core was six miles from the centre of Christchurch, 185 people were killed and the city was devastated. The quake and its numerous aftershocks were followed by liquefaction, the ground spewing up water and silty earth. Roads sank like whirlpools; hard rock, stone, tarmac and concrete became liquid. Whole streets of nineteenth-century wooden houses were destroyed, pavements and roads opened up and rubble, pipes and wiring, the innards of a modern city, came to the surface, like broken bones piercing skin. Christchurch looked as though it had been bombed.

Floods wreaked further havoc in the suburbs, where there were rockfalls and landslides, bent railway lines and houses teetering on newly created cliff tops. Fields on the edge of the city opened up huge deep gashes as they split apart. Aftershocks rippled across the land for months, including a series in December, just after I arrived in the country, ten months after the quake. There could be no reassurance that the earthquakes were over.

New Zealand is on the Pacific Ring of Fire, a geologically active region of shifting plates and volcanoes. The country experiences around 20,000 quakes a year, usually several hundred strong enough to feel, and it has a quake of six or more magnitude annually. In a country nicknamed the Shaky Isles, people know they live in an active quake zone, but the level of destruction of Christchurch shocked the nation to the core.

We're approaching Christmas now, and many of the pilots who have come to fly during the holidays live and work in Christchurch. When I meet them at the Kahu and out on the airfield, it is obvious that they are resilient but reeling, the psychological aftershocks of the quake rumbling on through them. Coming to fly in Omarama is a blessed relief, for many, from the tortuous processes of trying to rebuild their lives as well as their city, endless negotiations about insurance, and the uncertainty, the not knowing.

I talk to Terry Delore, a highly respected extreme endurance glider pilot. Terry was hang-gliding world champion in the 1970s, aged just seventeen, and now he is a legend in free flight. Gifted and determined, he has broken twenty-eight world records and flown over 2,500 kilometres in fifteen hours in the New Zealand wave; at the time, it was the longest soaring flight ever achieved.

Terry vividly recounts the day of the quake to me, watching his house ripple up and down as he stood in the road outside. A man with a phenomenal capacity to endure risk and the unknown, the impact of the earthquake on his city has shocked him. Terry is someone who is highly experienced at coping with the chaos and unpredictability of the natural world – in fact, he has learned to use them to do incredible things – so it is unnerving, though totally understandable, to see how unmoored he was by the earthquake.

Jenny Wilkinson lives in Christchurch and comes to fly at Omarama when she can get away. She has achieved a women's world record in gliding and has flown 1,000 kilometres in seven hours and seven minutes. As we talk, Jenny explains how the unpredictable, powerful, quickly changing sky seems more solid to her now than the land, which could erupt at any moment, creating whirlpools and holes where there had been solid earth.

'I feel safer and more in control at 18,000 feet without an engine than on the land,' she says.

The unstable sky has become a place of purchase for Jenny. We search for solid ground only to find that it's not available, that all is groundlessness.

As celebrations for the holidays continue, the campsite fills up, spilling over with brightly coloured tents and caravans. There's an unusual mix of people: some are from military flying careers, fighter pilots or commercial passenger-jet pilots, whose original passion for flying finds little expression in their professional work.

Trevor Mollard has captained passenger jets for many years, and he tells me that jet flying is about not making any mistakes. 'You plough through the air and avoid anything that might disrupt you. It's the repetition of standard procedures. Being creative and thinking on your feet is actively discouraged. You're operating a machine,' he says, 'the air is minor, but in gliding there is no machine; there's only the sky.'

Gliding keeps Trevor's love of flying alive and it's become an extension of him. 'Glider pilots talk about their flying in the first person,' he tells me. 'They say, "I turned", "I flew", "I caught the wave". You project yourself into the air and don't even think about what your hands and feet are doing, where the wings are. It becomes as natural as walking, even though building that mental picture of what's going on in the atmosphere is a major mental exercise.'

There are few environments in which fighter pilots and nature-loving sky surfers gladly mix, but this is one of them. Everyone here is searching for a deeper relationship with the elements, with the mountains and the skies that surround them.

As I spend more time getting to know the pilots at Omarama, I begin to see which pilots don't share their stories and just fly off on their own, seeking out the solitary release from society by disappearing into the mountains. Hiroko, a Japanese anaesthetist, comes to Omarama for a week, several times a season, hires Gavin's single-seat Discus and flies solo. Soaring here must be the exact opposite of anaesthesia, so perhaps that's why she loves it.

But I so enjoy hearing people's stories of their flights. At the end of a week, and with Gavin's mountain soaring course complete, the pilots at Omarama seem overwhelmed. Exhausted, stunned and amazed, each evening they laugh and talk in the Kahu before collapsing into bed in one of the airfield-side chalets or local hotels, dreaming of mountains and surging air masses.

Terry Duncan and Neita Montague are two visiting U.S. pilots from the Women Soaring Pilots Association, an organization that seeks to promote women in gliding. 'I've learned more here in one week,' says Terry, 'than I would have in several years, back in Nevada.'

At the end of a baking hot afternoon, a few days before Christmas, a cool sea breeze blows in from the east coast, turning the evening chilly. We have plans to go to the annual 'Bark Up' competition at the local pub in Omarama, so I pull on a warm jumper and hat before setting off with Bo and Pipe. Huddled in the crowd around the bar, a Speight's beer in my hand and the glass eye of a bull's stuffed head staring down at me, I gaze, along with everyone else in the pub, at a pool table in the centre of the room. It is covered by a board with a piece of red living-room carpet laid on top. Everyone is waiting. Finally, a man shuffles in through the pub's sliding side-door astride a ram, holding its curly horns. With the help of another man, they haul the creature on to the pool table, and the man who brought the ram in hops up on to the table and begins shearing it with old-fashioned hand shears. As the pop music blares and the chatter rumbles, he works deftly, manoeuvring the ram on to its side, its back, its other side, holding on to a sharp horn with one hand as the dusty grey merino fleece falls on to the red carpet, revealing that it's pure white underneath.

The opening ceremony of the Bark Up complete, the main event begins. Farmers take turns to bring in their noisiest huntaway sheepdogs, which they've trained to bark at sheep and cattle. Each baffled-looking dog is hupped on to the pool table and then its owner whistles. The idea is that the dogs bark in response, but some just look blankly at their whistling masters and stand on the table, wagging in silence. Others leap straight down off the table and run out of the side door. One big dark-brown dog stands amid the loud hum of people and blaring music, wagging and barking loudly, head turned upwards, before the enthusiastic applause sends him scurrying off. Another raises his head and barks into the air, turns and barks at the crowd and then turns again to bark at his owner. All the while, three judges sit stony-eyed on stools on the other side of the pool table, making notes on clipboards. I have no idea what criteria they are looking for.

After ten or so dogs, there is a lull before the winner is announced to raucous cheering and more delighted barking from the dog in question. The dog's name and that of its owner will be added to the list of Bark Up winners on the board on the pub wall.

*

During the holiday week, I feel far from home, but comforted by the various musician pilots who entertain us in the Kahu. Ricco, an Italian pilot who settled in New Zealand's North Island after years of living at sea, plays the cuatro, a large ukulele, and explains the dark story of why he was always destined to become a glider pilot: he was named after his Uncle Ricco, who died in a gliding accident in Switzerland the day before his nephew was born. On another evening Gerrard Dale, known simply as 'G', plays the piano accompanied by Sheena, a pilot from Queenstown, on her violin.

On Christmas Day itself, Dagmar serves a full Christmas dinner with all the trimmings for the whole of Gavin's crew and anyone who wants to join them. We sit at a long table, feasting in thirty-degree heat, and though I'm still a little homesick, it's a day of contentment and calm, with G playing the piano long into the evening.

Later, I speak with my family over Skype. They are together, having Christmas on the farm. I tell them I am growing salad rocket in tubs and hear my ninety-year-old grandmother in the background saying, in a voice filled with horror, 'Oh, no! She's not going up in a rocket now, is she?' I get a sudden insight into what she thinks I am doing: she seems to think that I've run away with the circus to the other side of the world to be shot out of a cannon!

Having watched and listened to G on the piano, I'm keen to ask him about his relationship with music. As I have learned to fly, as it has established itself in my life, I have wondered about how each flight is a musical experience of sorts — unsung, unwritten, except in the moment of flight. We draw musical notes in the sky as we twist and turn, climb and descend, and as my confidence has grown, soaring has become a kind of sky dancing: an intelligent connection between the glider and my body, and between the wings of the glider and the air around them. There is an architectural quality to flying that I recognize as musical, as though we're all parts of one vast orchestra.

G is a world-class glider pilot and one of Gavin's top instructors, but he's also a classically trained pianist, and there are some fascinating connections between his flying and his playing.

'They're both a lifetime's work,' he says. Like playing the piano, 'You can fly gliders forever; most serious glider pilots I know will not stop flying until they run out of life.' G takes a swig of red wine and goes on. 'One thing they have in common is that they're both, on the face of it, really logical, straightforward wheels-and-gears occupations, scientific — except, that's only a part of it. Both of them,' he continues, 'have a whole other side, which is hard to define . . . I call it "non-linear". Stuff happens when you play the piano and fly gliders . . . It's to do with character, emotion and chance.'

I think of Bo, and how he plays his glider like an instrument, like it is an extension of himself; climbing inside and setting off into the sky, he is like a musician chasing a melody. Like mastering an instrument, soaring requires a scientific understanding of the discipline, precision, hours and hours of practice, and total, passionate commitment.

I ask G to compare playing a piece of music with soaring.

'Flying is different in that you respond to what the air tells you, so there's more give and take between you and the medium. You're not trying to do the same thing every time. But, fundamentally, you're trying to produce the perfect shining flight . . . and flying, like music, is all about rhythm.' He explains this further: 'There's a rhythm to a successful flight,' he says. 'It flows. It bounces. It's like when you run across a stream bed. You jump from rock to rock, and you can't stop on any one rock long enough, because you will fall in the water if you do. But, if you bounce from rock to rock, you don't get wet. That constant movement through the sky is analogous to the constant movement through time in a piece of music. In flying, we even use the word "rhythm".' He pauses for a moment, then adds, 'There's something beautiful, something really lovely in making the aircraft move through the sky in the right place, a purity of line.'

He compares teaching flying and the piano, too: 'Words don't work for music and it's the same when you feel the air; words are too slow, too linear.'

A few weeks ago, I went to one of G's daily talks on gliding in the Southern Alps. In the talk, he broke down into bite-size lessons what he has made instinctive through years of dedication to free flight, but I could see that he couldn't quite express the rapture of gliding in words. Instead, he drew diagrams on the whiteboard, focused on the practical business of the changing conditions; how to

turn in the core of a thermal, how to recognize a convergence; katabatic winds, orographic clouds – the difference
between maintaining attitude – the angle of the nose; and
maintaining speed, how to read the flow of air around the
mountains and valleys, and the intricacies of the wave. And
what he didn't say, he expressed through his body. He
stood up, wielding a model glider, both arms out. He flew
around the room, reliving thermals, rotor, stalls and spins
– re-experiencing the drama of the sky.

As a total beginner, much of what G said went over my
head, so I watched him instead. I almost wanted to block
my ears, to focus on what his body was saying underneath
the talk of rates of climb, trends in the vario and final
glide. His movements so clearly showed his passion for
flying.

If the skill of successful soaring is akin to that of playing
a musical instrument, then the experience of unpowered
flight also shares something with music. Both can be
bone-shaking experiences, both can transform you inter-
nally. They are emergent, emotional. I remember being
told I would sing on my first solo flight, and I can imagine
why one might only be able to express the euphoria of the
sky with music.

*

It is early January and I haven't flown for several weeks
because the Glide Omarama team have been so busy over
the holiday season. I feel frustrated, landlocked, lonely for
the sky. I am suffering from low-altitude sickness. There've

been several non-flyable days, now, with clouds stuck on the top of the mountains, keeping us all grounded, held under, and there is an air of restlessness at Omarama as pilots pace about, gazing upwards. Our community is shot through with cabin fever.

Then, a few days later, the weather changes. I meet Justin, Gavin's cousin, at the Kahu; his client for the day hasn't shown up, so he is free to fly with me. It is twenty-eight degrees, a difficult, windy, blue thermal day, with no cumulus clouds marking the lift. These conditions are too tough for me, so Justin will do all the flying, but I'm excited nonetheless, uncertain what to expect.

We set off, climb in the Nursery Ridge thermals, and then drop low and I think we'll have to turn back and land. The weight of disappointment sinks in my stomach at the thought. But Justin is quiet, concentrating on the feel of the invisible air, and slowly we edge up the side of Horrible to 6,000 feet and out across the Mackenzie Basin, over to Magic and the Diadems. The heat and glare of the sun are remorseless, and this, combined with the movement of the glider, makes me feel nauseous. I find that it helps to put my right hand on the stick very gently as Justin moves it subtly this way and that, forward and back.

We enter the Barrier Range, head due north and, for the first time, I fly into the Alps proper. We are surrounded on every side; all I see above and around me are sharp, steep, vertical, jagged, bony rocks, covered in ice. I've the feeling of being inside the mountains. We soar low on ridge lift and then Justin circles and climbs in a thermal to rise up over the peaks, then we descend again and fly up close to the mountain face. I stare up at the dark-grey rocks, spotted with white ice, small glaciers picking out the shapes of the gullies in which they're frozen.

A peace descends inside the cockpit. Justin's flying is smooth, with no sharp movements or hard edges, and he exudes a calm confidence. If he is reserved on the ground, the potential danger of the situation peels all that away up here. He points out favourite mountains and valleys and land-out options, and I'm utterly engrossed in the moment, alert with fascination as great sharp mountains fly past at our wing tip. There's an odd mismatch between the space we are flying in and the atmosphere inside the cockpit, a stark contrast between worlds just a few inches apart. Outside are jagged rocks, howling winds and looming glacial crevasses, but, in here, all is tranquil.

Justin takes a thermal, we bank and circle with the rocky horizon sliding past. The mountain ridge flies up vertically in my view as we tip on to our side. I look down at a tarn of glacial melt, high up in the mountains. It's a big blue eye staring up at us. We drop lower and the rocks loom overhead again, tall peaks way above us. I gaze up at them as we fly, sculling amongst the rocks, crags and glaciers slicing the mountainside, falling in slow motion. As Justin banks and wheels, the rocks twist and move about us. We fly directly at peaks and then edge around the side of them.

This is a familiar flight for Justin, but it's my first into the higher Alps, my first experience of intimacy with the big mountains. I have to remind myself that we're flying in energy created by these bodies of rock. The sky and mountains are in great conversation, embroiled in a dynamic, explosive interaction; those rocks are dangerous, but it's their volatile, passionately unstable relationship with the air around them that creates the lift.

We head towards Mount Brewster, a triangular peak rearing up out of a glacier that descends in rippling waves of ice all the way down the side of the mountain. We fly towards the glacier-encrusted rock, and it grows larger in my view, filling the whole cockpit as we descend. Justin points out a tiny black dot on the flat region of the glacier. 'A geologist,' he says. Then he drops the nose unexpectedly, taking me aback, and we dive and descend fast towards the figure, to skim over the icy terrain. My thighs tense and, heart thumping, I shuffle in my seat, pushing back against my parachute.

As we fly beyond the glacier, around the side of Mount Brewster's rocky summit, the mountain becomes sharper and more pointed before it softens and rounds out. The mountains are solid, imposing, immovable, but from the air they seem to shift, so it's impossible to say what overall shape they really are. The Southern Alps are like some giant unknowable body.

This perception is written into the Maori landscape-creation mythology. The first people here named the sky, land, forests and oceans as gods, and the entire landscape is imbued with ancestral myth that blurs the boundaries between humans and the rest of the land and its animals. Many mountains are mythic characters turned to stone. Aoraki is named after one of several brothers who arrived by canoe, back in the mythological past; the South Island is said to be their wrecked canoe, the highest peak of the Southern Alps its upturned hull, on which Aoraki (sometimes given as Aorangi) stood. The volcanic mountains of the North Island, Taranaki and Tongariro, are restless warriors who fought over a maiden. The origin of Lake Wakatipu, south-west of Omarama, near Queenstown, is explained in the story of the body of a giant named Matau, who kidnapped a Maori woman called Manata and kept her trapped in the mountains. She was rescued by her lover, Matakauri, who set fire to the sleeping giant. The burnt imprint of his body in the ground became the lake. The lake's water rises and falls most days, and that is said to be caused by the pulsating heart of the giant that lies, still beating, at the bottom of the lake.

*

Perhaps the last remnant of the ancient reverence for mountains as the realm of gods and mythology surfaced in the European naming of mountains after body parts. The mountains here have ribs and spines, there's Backbone Peak, the Tooth, Breast Hill, Chest Peak, the Two Thumbs Range, the Tusk – as though the mountains are the giant dismembered body of a fallen god. If this is fanciful, flying on the energetic lift created by the mountains re-enchants them; the dead materialism of my secular imagination is

lifted momentarily, suspended, as I'm suspended, travelling almost one hundred miles per hour amid the rocks.

We fly over the Haast Pass and look down on to tem-
perate rainforest, Alpine glaciers reaching into the trees
and almost to the sea. Justin points out that we're flying
along the 'main divide' of the Southern Alps. On one side,
the water flows to the east; on the other side, it flows to
the west.

We head north, towards Mount Sefton, before reaching what glider pilots call 'The Wall', a steep cliff of a
mountain that, on this thermal and ridge day, blocks our
path. In the distance, thirty kilometres away, I see a white
triangle reaching above everything else. It's my first
glimpse of Mount Cook, huge and tantalizing because we
can't reach it.

*

I don't have to worry about controlling the glider today,
and so I find I am moving in and out of an almost trance-
like state, quietly absorbing the extraordinary land and sky
all around me. Flying like this makes me feel that everything I went through with the illness was worthwhile,
because it got me to this place. I have never experienced
anything so extraordinary. Learning to fly is like asking the
universe a question: asking it to let me go into the world
to live and soar with joy and the possibility of death. It is
to ask to be graced with grace, filled with emptiness, to
arrive and never arrive. Flying brings you into greater
intimacy with nature. That's what I've been searching for,

up here. The natural world can hold any hurt inside it, recognize it, gently turn it over in the palm of its hand like a precious stone, and I have the sense now that the sky has crept up into my spine, worked its blue way into my bones.

We turn on to the Neumann Range and fly south. I look down on the Hopkins River, and over to the other side, to the Dobson River, flowing to join the head of Lake Ohau. We gain some altitude to cross on to the Ben Ohau Range, beginning our return leg to Omarama. Soaring over a mountain pass is tricky; Justin approaches alongside the pass and flies parallel with it, so he can either turn away, if we get into sink or rough air, or turn towards it and fly across on to the other side. The air is good, and we manoeuvre smoothly over the pass to the other side of the mountain range.

Once over the pass, we fly out of the bony outcrops of the Alpine peaks to a softer landscape that rolls down into a flat-bottomed valley. I look over to Lake Pukaki, which is a light, bright blue and quite different to the other lakes in the area due to the minerals washed into the water from the Tasman glacier, up in the Alps. Where the river merges into the lake, dark blue blends into light.

I take over and fly us back to Omarama on the final glide, spiralling down and on to the landing circuit.

'You have good control,' comments Justin, as the glider slows to a stop. 'I think you're ready to fly solo.'

I beam.

It's early evening and I've the thrilling feeling of having

visited another planet, one where there's only sky and rock and ice. The four hours of my flight with Justin are huge in my memory, a period of time 9,000 feet high. As I walk across the airfield, I'm almost shaking, partly with hunger, partly with a sense of having been blown open by that flight.

A few days ago, I watched a pilot land on his own for the first time. As he stepped out of the glider, he removed his trainers and knelt, head bowed, on the dry grass in front of a group of his friends as they emptied buckets of ice-cold water over his blond head. He was being baptized by his fellow junior glider pilots, initiated into the soaring fraternity.

Going solo for the first time in a glider is a big moment in a pilot's life – a real turning point. It's not something I want to do – whilst I am here, I want to be in the midst of the mountains, not circling repeatedly above an airfield – but I am glowing with pride that Justin thinks I could fly alone, and that jubilance lasts and lasts. I jog to one of the bikes leaning against the wall of Gavin's office, scoop it up and pedal furiously to the end of the airfield and back, burning some of the joy off.

That evening, at the Kahu, I find myself raving about the day's flight to anyone who will listen. I loved the feeling of pushing further into the terrain, of exploring a place humans cannot inhabit. Here was the sublime that mountains are known to offer, something more than beauty – a sense of power, of being imminently over-whelmed and swallowed up. Despite Justin's composure, it had felt like the rocks might reach out and grab us at any moment. When I say that, Bo nods: 'On average, one person dies every year in a gliding accident here.' We fall silent.

Chapter Twelve

Breathing at Altitude

A map of the Southern Alps is projected on to a screen in the briefing room. The contours of the landscape are shown in thin red lines that look like veins and blood vessels, brain-like in the way they wind and weave and fold back upon one another. The shapes of nature repeat themselves. It's an MRI scan of the mountains.

In each morning meeting, Gavin's team of instructors debrief the previous day's flights with students on the Mountain Soaring Course using SeeYou software linked to GPS devices in the gliders to create graphic representations of each flight. Someone dims the lights and closes the blind on the searing sun and then whole flights are played back, paused, rewound and played again, the tiny glider symbol moving over the digital map on the wall. We can see each circling thermal taken and the detailed contours of the flights along ridges and wave bars of lift.

Instructors dissect each flight, analysing what happened and why, and talk about how the country 'behaves', as though it were alive. They're like a group of doctors gathered to examine a projection of a brain scan. Even after a flight of several hours, covering hundreds of kilometres, up to high altitudes, these pilots look for ways it could have been improved. There's a sense of the infinite amount there is to learn about soaring. It's bottomless. 'You can't hope to get to the end of it in one lifetime,' says Trevor Mollard; even the experts are still learning, honing, deepening their understanding of how these mountains shape the fantastically unstable air around them.

*

Later that afternoon, Lemmy Tanner, one of Gavin's instructors, offers to fly with me. Lemmy is British, but spends the southern summers flying with Gavin's team. He learned to fly gliders as a teenager, in the 1950s, and stayed at the flying school at the weekends, working at the airfield in exchange for launches, before entering the R.A.F. on a scholarship. Across his flying career, he's flown a huge range of planes, including Tiger Moths, Austers, Jet Provosts, Vampires, Canberras, Victor tankers, Chipmunks and Varsities. His real flying passion is for soaring, though. As we tow up, he admits that, when he was younger, to be airborne was a chance to be away from the stresses on the ground. 'It used to be an escape mechanism,' he says, 'from people . . . the aggro.'

Lemmy takes us up to cloud base in thermals, letting me fly when we're in the lift, and suddenly we hit rotor turbulence. I know that strong turbulence can exist below wave lift, but I haven't yet experienced it in any real strength, and its power comes as a shock. The cumulus clouds above our heads look soft and insubstantial, but that belies the rough, strong energy they harbour. They are torn, rolling over on themselves, shredded by the wave just above the cumulus layer. We must push on through the rotor to get to the smooth wave lift above.

The glider rumbles up and down, the wings wobble and bounce. I'm rattled around in my seat, my heart beating faster. I ask Lemmy to take over, and look ahead at the white rippling horizon of the Southern Alps and down at the dry, brown back of the Ewe Range as we jolt in the rough air. Lemmy finds a hole in the cumulus layer and we begin to rise up, still being thrown about. I'm not exactly uncomfortable, but I am aware of my situation in a way I haven't been before: here I am, at 8,000 feet, strapped into an engineless plane, being rattled and jarred in powerful turbulence. The air around us feels thick, both familiar and foreign. It won't let me fall, I remind myself.

As we pump through the rotor, Lemmy is unperturbed; he has complete faith in the glider's ability to withstand the rough air. He didn't warn me about the rotor because he's used to flying with experienced soaring pilots. It would be like reassuring someone that a bumpy track is safe in an S.U.V. His indifference leaves me feeling out of my depth, which, of course, I am.

'It's just air,' he says. But he admits that it's powerful. 'Mountains produce the most changeable, dynamic air and the most varied conditions for free flight,' he says. 'There's tremendous energy in the atmosphere around mountains and it's far more volatile than people think. When you walk around on the ground, the air isn't any great resistance, but when you're doing sixty knots, it's substantial.'

As we bounce upwards, I remember what G told me: he pictures a glider in rotor as a child's rattle. No matter how hard you shake it, it will not break and the beads will not fall out. His description is reassuring, but only to a point.

The glider is thrown this way and that, and then suddenly we push up through the cumulus layer, like a cork popping up through water. Lemmy has made contact with the wave; we're on the rising front of it and ascending fast. The turbulence has completely disappeared and soon I'm looking down on the clouds. The landscape is big and layered, the white line of the Alps on the horizon mirrored by the cumulus clouds above, a ghostly reflection of the mountains, floating in the air.

It was worth pushing through the rotor to get to this and, as the alarm that surfaced in me is smoothed away by the silken wave, I take hold of the stick and put my feet back on the rudder pedals. The blue sky dominates my view as I fly straight and level along the wave line, continuing to steadily gain altitude. As we speed higher and higher, the altimeter needle hits ten knots, the maximum rate of climb it can register, and stays there, pressed against the end of the dial. I've no idea how fast we're ascending.

When we reach 9,000 feet, the audio vario beeping fast and high-pitched, Lemmy tells me to lean forward and turn on the oxygen, get the cannula out of the side pocket and place it around my face, over my ears and clip the feed under my nose. The transparent plastic tube trails behind my head, back towards the oxygen canister stowed behind Lemmy in the fuselage. He puts a cannula on too. The glider has a regulated-demand oxygen system that follows the rhythm of my own breath, blowing oxygen up my nose every time I breathe in and stopping when I breathe out, to prevent wastage. I've the odd feeling of being breathed by the machine.

Now, in addition to the deep howl of the air outside and the beeping of the audio vario inside, we have the gentle puffing noise of the oxygen system breathing with us. It adds an organic sound to the interior of the cockpit, further blurring the boundary between our bodies and the aircraft. One bleeds into the other, biology is extended, machine is embodied.

Lemmy has felt connected to his glider from early on in his soaring. 'I used to think, I'm just like a bird,' he says. 'The glider is the shell, the body of the bird, and I am . . . I am . . .' He cannot find the words. 'You become part of it,' he adds. That sensation is part of becoming an experienced glider pilot. 'If you can get to that stage, you can manoeuvre the glider anywhere you want to. Rather than thinking about how to control the machine you're sitting in, you think, This is all part of me,' says Lemmy.

I push back into my parachute and spread my hand against the body of the glider. We're a big, breathing, soaring bird.

Lemmy has had some memorable encounters with birds in wave. Bird strike is a real danger for powered planes, can wreck a jet engine or propeller, but, when soaring without an engine, it's possible to fly close to birds safely, if they will permit you. Soaring at 12,000 feet, in autumn wave, in Scotland, Lemmy came across a skein of Canada geese, flying in formation, west, above the cumulus cloud layer. Birds know how to use the winds to conserve energy, not only in soaring on ridge and thermal lift, but also on lee-wave systems, using the power in the sky for their long migrations. They've long known how to use the complex workings of the atmospheric wave that we're only just beginning to understand, so when you are in a glider, hunting for lift, and see birds soaring, it's always wise to follow them.

The best kind of simplicity, so they say, is on the other side of complicated, and that's where we are with modern gliders, highly engineered to a perfect pure design. It makes it hard to understand why it took humans so long to work out how to soar. We never needed an engine. Why, Lemmy asks, couldn't people have looked at soaring birds and seen that you can fly without flapping?

'I still can't work it out,' he goes on. 'Over the centuries, people weren't able to devise even a little tiny paper model that would fly. If they had gone to a cliff top with the wind blowing up it and watched the birds soaring, and if they'd only realized the way the birds were flying, they could probably have come up with a lightweight wood model.' Lemmy develops a counter-narrative of human history in which soaring flight was invented thousands of years ago.

I admit that I've puzzled over this. We managed to build canoes, boats, rafts and sailing ships that crossed the oceans on the winds. Since we had lightweight wood, rope and glues, we could have developed man-carrying gliders with the ability to soar on the winds as birds do, just as we are now.

The Maori have a long tradition of making kites. These manu tukutuku ('manu' means both kite and bird; 'tuku-tuku' refers to the unwinding of the string as the kite lifts higher) are central to Maori religion and mythology, and were a way to communicate with the gods, Maui, Rangi and Tane. They were also used for divination, particularly in the event of war. A priest would fly a kite and read the way it moved through the air. Kites were also flown to celebrate the Maori New Year, when the constellation Pleiades, known as Matariki, appeared in a certain spot in the winter night sky. Many Maori kites were made as figures of people with outstretched arms, their cloaks taking on the shape of wings. Old Maori texts talk of giant kites, which apparently took ten, twenty, even thirty men to send up and manipulate with strings. These kites were surely large and strong enough to carry a man aloft, so it's hard to understand why a culture with at least 1,000 years of kite flying didn't try to attach a man to one.

But, until Lilienthal and the Wrights, several thousand years after the invention of the kite, we just didn't see the potential of soaring flight on fixed wings (although there are some tales of man-carrying kites in ancient China).

'Watching birds of prey or seabirds soaring should have

given people more of a clue,' Lemmy goes on, frustration in his voice. He sounds almost angry that it took us so long to work it out; I can feel him imagining all the time that's been lost looking up at the sky.

We've reached 12,000 feet and, while it's thirty degrees on the ground, up here, it is well below freezing. I'm wearing jeans, flip-flops and a long-sleeved T-shirt. I'm hardly dressed for the cold and my feet begin to freeze, but, as we bank, the piercing sun shines momentarily on them, providing some relief. I wiggle my toes.

Peering down through the cloud layer, I can make out that we're over the Hawkdun Range, to the south of Omarama. The cumulus layer has grown and changed beneath us, and now covers much of the ground. We will have to find holes in the cloud to get back down.

We fly fifty kilometres to Lake Ohau and reach a gap in the clouds. Through it, I can see the glint of the Ahuriri River, a thin, grey pencil-squiggle, from 13,000 feet. I take over and fly at sixty knots along the invisible wave, until we reach the part of the wave that is going down and we fly into nine-knot sink. Like an ocean wave, wave lift always has a side flowing upward and a side flowing downward, and Lemmy tells me to speed up to ninety knots to get through it and into the next area of lift. The sound of the air gets much louder as I dip the nose and speed up, the audio vario howling to tell us what we already know: that we're losing altitude fast. We progress and find the next upward-moving air; I bring the nose up, slow down and continue along the wave, ascending once again.

Then Omarama base comes on the radio and calls
Lemmy back for a flying lesson. We descend through a
hole in the clouds, their edges touching either wing,
enveloping us briefly; we bounce around in the rotor and
descend some more. Lake Ohau grows larger as we spiral
down and fly back to Omarama.

As Lemmy and I clamber out of the cockpit, I find
myself thanking him enthusiastically, still high from the
flight. The skill and subtlety involved in wave flying, the
ability to feel out the air around the glider, are astound-
ing and, though the rotor turbulence was disconcerting,
I am already itching to work my way back through it to
the wave above, to soar higher still. From 13,000 feet, the
world looked so different, the landscape I am just getting
to know appeared totally new.

Later that afternoon, I am still feeling taut and heightened, so when Bo says he is going down to the riverbank
to shoot the plastic milk bottles he has been collecting, I
find myself leaping at the chance to go with him. Bo and
I drive down to the riverbank, armed with a .22 rifle, a
.410 shotgun, a twelve-gauge pump-action shotgun with
the end sawn off, and all of his milk bottles, filled with
water. We line the bottles up at the bottom of the bank,
so that, if we miss, the bullets will go straight into the
earth. I press the .22 rifle into my right shoulder, focus on
a bottle through the eye piece, hold my breath and pull the
trigger. The butt of the gun punches hard against my
shoulder and the cartridge explodes, piercing numerous
holes in the bottle, which gushes out water. I'm reminded

of Emily Dickinson's poem, 'My Life has stood – a Loaded Gun' as I sit back on my heels, steady my breathing, and take aim again.

*

Over the next few days, I talk with several pilots about New Zealand's famous wave. I want to understand it better, even if I'll never learn to recognize it in the sky. Justin tells me, 'Reading a wave sky is a fine art,' and Bo draws endless diagrams on a whiteboard to explain the science behind it, but I remain puzzled, my sky literacy still poor.

The full potential of wave flying hasn't yet been reached, and the US Perlan Project, named after the mother-of-pearl clouds that have been spotted at very high altitudes, aims to fly a glider to 90,000 feet in wave, to explore the way in which the rippling air that forms in the lee of big mountains rises into the stratosphere. The Perlan Project's first attempt to reach great heights was based in Omarama in the early 2000s. Former U.S. Air Force and N.A.S.A. test pilot Einar Enevoldson and adventurer Steve Fossett launched from the airfield in a normal glider, wearing astronauts' pressure suits. Though they didn't get as high as they had hoped, they later flew in wave formed in the lee of the Argentinian Andes and gained the current glider altitude record of 50,722 feet, way above the height at which passenger jets can fly.

The project is now building a pressurized glider to aim even higher. The thin air at very high altitude will mean that it will have to fly at high speed, over 350 knots, and will fly close to what's known as the 'coffin corner', where there's very little wriggle room between the stall speed (too slow) and the maximum speed the aircraft can safely perform.

Justin Wills tells me that he thinks the future of wave flying could be in exploring the jet stream. Gliders, he thinks, might be able to use the wave to fly up into the jet stream to circumnavigate vast distances across the planet. What an extraordinary thought: a plane crossing the planet with no interior source of energy.

*

Now that I'm embarking on longer, higher cross-country flights, I need to make sure I keep hydrated by drinking plenty of water. So I also need to face the problem of how to pee in flight. For men, this is a bit simpler. Many pilots don't even have to let go of the stick to pee into bio-degradable plastic bags that they fling out of the air vent. Others simply wear incontinence diapers. I don't like the idea of sitting in a wet nappy, but there's hardly another option for women. I laugh about the issue with Bo, whose face darkens. 'It really is a problem,' he says. 'You have to keep hydrated to ensure clear thinking. If you're up there for hours under a hot sun, you will get dehydrated if you don't drink.' And a full bladder can be distracting, can draw focus and prevent concentration. He's annoyed with my flippancy and, feeling chastened, I try to wipe the smirk off my face.

The next day, I find myself hovering outside a pharmacy in Twizel, my fingers on the door handle, too embarrassed to go in and ask for a packet of incontinence pads. My physical dignity only recently restored after my treatment, I resist, but Bo pushes past me, strides in and comes out moments later with a packet of huge padded diapers. I wonder if the pharmacy is used to glider pilots buying them.

Thankfully, women pilots are seeking solutions elsewhere, and I meet with a few of Omarama's visiting female pilots to discuss the issue. The answer, it seems, is a silicon contraption that I can only describe as a rubber imprint of a vagina with a narrow cup sticking out of it like a beckoning forefinger. I'm reminded of the contraceptive nurse showing me a rubber cap, many years ago. The cup inserts like a tampon and sits beneath the urethra, collecting the urine and sending it down the rubber tube attached to a collecting bag. Developed by Katrin Senne, a champion German glider pilot and doctor, it's a bit like an advanced Shewee, but is designed to be worn sitting down. The contraption has allowed women to double the length of their flights. I put in an order.

*

A few weeks later, mine arrives, along with several bags with tubes that connect to the rubber finger at the end of the silicon cup, which is soft and dark pink. The instructions say to pee gently to avoid leakage and suggest wearing an incontinence pad as well; the device should be washed by putting it in a 'cleaning bath for false teeth.'

Bo warns me that it's surprisingly difficult to persuade yourself to pee in flight and says that some people practise by sitting in an empty bath wearing an adult diaper and drink several litres of water until they have to go. He suggests I practise, but I don't listen; I am keen to get up into the air with my new device.

I have the opportunity a few days later. It is a warm mid-February day, Bo has an afternoon free and there's a spare glider in the fleet. He looks up at the sky, towards the Alps, and says, 'Wave is happening.' He checks the oxygen supply, anticipating altitude.

This time, I prepare. I wear thick merino-wool socks, hiking boots, warm tracksuit bottoms, incontinence knickers that come almost up to my waist, a fleece, a sunhat and a scarf. It's hot and I'm overdressed, but I'm not thinking about the ground. I'm dressed for altitude.

I go to the bathroom at the airfield and insert the silicon device, attaching it to a rubber tube that goes down the inside of my trousers. It's designed to be worn sitting, not walking, and I waddle across the airfield to the launch point, my legs slightly apart. I picture Amy Johnson and Amelia Earhart pointing at me and laughing.

We take off, I do the long aerotow and we release over the Nursery Ridge. Bo takes us up in ridge lift, then in thermals south-west to the Lindis Range, or 'Okahu' in Maori – place of the kahu hawk. Soon, we reach the rotor beneath the cloud layer and rock and rumble in it as Bo concentrates on locating the parts of the tumbling turbulence that are moving up, so we can use them as a staircase to the wave above. I find I am tensing in the rough air, but we quickly pass through the rotor and wind along the wave, climbing and heading north into the Alps.

I take over and feel the silken lift, though I still can't read the wave bars. The sky is a chaotic mass of cloud layers to me. Below is the lumpy cumulus layer, ripped by the wave, and, high above us, the thick lenticular clouds are stacked like a pile of pancakes with the smooth texture of softly whisked egg white. This is the most complex sky I've ever flown in, a mix of cumulus, stratus whipped into lenticulars, alto stratus, and winds at different speeds, blowing in different directions. These clouds have become another layer of landscape, a cloudscape – not castles, but mountains in the air.

We continue to climb, faster now, the audio vario almost a solid, high-pitched squeal. The hands on the altimeter dial wind like a clock in fast-forward, but for me time has slowed, almost stopped. We reach 10,000 feet; I switch on the oxygen and put on the cannula as we continue to ascend. We head on to the Maitland Ridge, fly up the Hopkins Valley, reach 15,000 feet and continue north over the Neumann Range. As we climb, the air pressure reduces, so Bo tells me to turn the oxygen flow up. I turn it up again at 18,000 feet. By the time we reach 20,000 feet, the bright blue lakes are visible in their entirety, and the ground, blurred and flattened into browns and greys and icy whites, seems to have shrunk away. The sky dominates my view.

I'm surrounded by transparent tubes that connect to various orifices, one from my nose into the instrument panel, where it connects with the oxygen-delivery system, another down my leg, from my urethra into a plastic bag. I'm using a cannula, bottled pure oxygen, incontinence knickers, an inflatable cushion designed for people sitting for long periods in wheelchairs and an external catheter – all apparatus normally associated with medical care. Until a few days ago, I hadn't seen a cannula since my year of hospitals, and I naturally associate it with illness, but here it's what enables us to fly higher, reach beyond the capacity of our bodies and take them to places they're not designed to go. This flying is the opposite of illness, made possible, paradoxically, by the very same technology.

I've been swigging water for the last two hours and can feel the pressure of a full bladder. Bo is flying, so I decide now is the time. Nothing happens. I try to make myself pee, but it's as ineffective as trying to force myself to go to sleep. Clearly, my brain has a deep-seated abhorrence of the idea of peeing in my pants. Potty training runs deep. I try again and again, but it doesn't work, and so I sit with a painfully full bladder, looking down at the clouds as we continue to fly towards Lake Pukaki. I'm 21,000 feet above the world, but have taken its bodily taboos up with me.

Flying above 20,000 feet brings a few other considerations too. At these altitudes, the instruments under-read due to the lower air pressure. We mustn't exceed the V.N.E. of the glider, the maximum airspeed, because it could make the ailerons flutter and endanger the airframe. Bo has a rule of thumb that the airspeed indicator under-reads by a percentage roughly equivalent to your altitude; so, here, at 21,000 feet, it will under-read by about twenty per cent. The V.N.E. is a red line on the dial, and, flying so high, we must keep away from it; I need my instruments uncovered now.

Flying at this altitude also means we have reached a danger zone in terms of hypoxia. With no time to acclimatize and having gone from 2,000 feet to 20,000 in under an hour, if our oxygen flow were to break down at this altitude, we'd have only a few minutes before we'd pass out. One of the many symptoms of hypoxia is euphoria. A book I borrowed a few weeks ago, called *Human Factors for Pilots*, says that one of the first signs of hypoxia is 'apparent personality change', characterized by 'a change in outlook and behaviour with euphoria and loss of inhibitions.' Now, staring out at this huge sky, I wonder if I'd even be able to recognize those signs of hypoxia. I always feel euphoric when I'm soaring, that's why I do it. Even now, desperate for the loo and with my bladder stubbornly refusing my brain's instructions, joy pulses through my chest as we bank in the wave.

Bo's way of staying alert to potential hypoxia is to keep an eye on our mental alertness and use that as a measure to ensure the oxygen flow is still working and that it's turned up enough. He asks me to say the alphabet backwards, not something I can do even on the ground, and he remains serious and quiet as I screw it up.

*

The cumulus layer, 10,000 feet below, begins to cover most of the ground and soon we're high above a white world. We reach 22,000 feet (four miles high) and fly right over the peak of Mount Cook, which just pierces through the clouds below. It's my second glimpse of 'the Rock', this time from above, but, again, surrounded on all sides by clouds that cover the rest of the 12,000-feet peaks, I cannot see it clearly.

The sun is piercing, so I cover my face, including my nose, with a white scarf. I'm completely hidden, apart from my hands. I bank and circle, some cloud clears and I peer down through the mist of thinned cumulus to the grey moraine of the Tasman Glacier, where it melts into Lake Tasman, which becomes a river that becomes another lake, Lake Pukaki, which is covered with the dark splotches of cloud shadows. The bright blue of Lake Pukaki shines up through the opaque cumulus. There's a distinct line where the braided river meets the lake waters; the lake seems to bloom out of the grey shale riverbed, so electric blue it looks artificial.

We are flying fast, the noise of the air almost drowning out the gentle puffs of the oxygen. By now, we're not far from the cruising altitude of passenger jets. I've a feeling of quiet triumph, but I'm also aware that we can't get down quickly. I can see Lakes Ohau, Pukaki and Tekapo all at the same time; the land has become coherent, but distant. Usually, when I fly, I feel connected to the landscape underneath me, but now that link feels broken and I have to remind myself that it's the mountains that are creating this wave lift. This is action at a distance, invisible and deferred, but I feel like a sailor, far out to sea, with no land visible on the horizon. We're cut off, remote from the ground.

At the southern end of the Ben Ohau Range, we must descend to 17,500 feet, due to airspace restrictions. Bo takes over and pulls out the air brakes, which make us descend quickly, and then I fly us back into the Mackenzie Basin, concentrating on the horizon ahead and not my painfully full bladder. Descending to 15,000, 10,000, 6,000 feet, we drop through the rotor (I grit my teeth), descend below the cumulus layer and there, again, are the Cloud Hills and Mount Benmore.

The wind has picked up since we left. The willow trees along the edge of the airfield are bent low, the windsock is horizontal and we have to do the landing fast, so as to maintain control in the turbulent wind on the ground. We roll along the grass, stop, I take off the cannula, lift open the canopy and climb out with my peeing contraption still attached. I stomp over to the edge of the airfield as best I can on rapidly thawing feet, to where the male glider pilots pee before they launch. I reach inside my tracksuit, pull out the end of the foot-long rubber tube, hold it and urinate standing up, my feet apart. It's an odd sensation to stand and pee like a man, and it gives me a momentary

thrill, a feeling of transgression. I watch the urine disappear into the dry tussock grass. I shake the tube when I'm
done and place it back inside my trousers. Amy Johnson,
Amelia Earhart and I throw our heads back and laugh.

*

A few days later, I arrive on the airfield to rumours circulating in the terminal building and the Kahu. Someone is
dead. Gavin and Bo stand talking by the aviation gas
pump outside the building, their heads bowed, staring at
the dust. An hour later, we all look up to watch a rescue
helicopter come in to land on the airfield with a white
glass-fibre coffin attached to one landing skid. There he is.
Michael McKellow, known as Joe, crashed. His friend had
been flying in another glider and watched helplessly as Joe
turned to the right, towards Snowy Top on the Diadem
Range, and, upside down, crashed at speed into the side
of it. Joe was dead when the rescue services reached the
site. The glider was shattered.

I find it hard to believe that there is now a blank space
where a man has recently been. Joe's things are in the
hangar. He was in the Kahu, chatting to Bo, this morning.
The risk and danger of soaring has always been theoretical
to me. I knew it was possible to die in a glider, but I didn't
really *know* it was possible. Now that it has happened, I am
in disbelief, overcome with sadness. How naive I was.

Emails and calls come through to pilots from friends
who have heard that someone has died out of Omarama.
The news reports the crash without naming the pilot;

Joe's son is in flight somewhere abroad, and the authorities want to wait until he lands and can be told in person before releasing the dead pilot's name to the press. I picture a shock wave chasing Joe's son through the air, ready to engulf him when he reaches the ground.

'It always happens this way,' says Bo, 'when they don't release the name.' And I realize properly for the first time that this has happened before, many times before. A side of gliding that I'd thus far refused to look at suddenly comes into focus and I'm forced to face the truth. This sport has serious dangers lurking in it.

The next morning, the weather briefing goes ahead as normal. At the end, Gavin makes a short speech about Joe before there is a minute's silence. We stand; some people close their eyes. Then the minute is over and everyone files out, ready to begin the day's flying. There is a sense of sorrow, but not of shock. Everyone is just carrying on. I can't work out if it's a form of denial or their way of dealing with their sadness, to get back out there and up into the sky.

The following day, Gavin chairs a meeting to discuss the crash and explore whether anything could have been done differently to prevent it, whether more flight-skill checks of visiting pilots are necessary. They conclude that nothing more could have been done. Joe's death was just one of those things.

A day or so later, while the wreckage of Joe's glider is still on the mountaintop, I have a local flying lesson with Bo. I fly along the Diadems and, as we pass Snowy Top, my

eye is drawn down to the flat, innocent-looking mountain.
Don't look down, I tell myself. Don't look. I can't see the
wreckage, but I picture it in my mind's eye and I can't help
but wonder if this mountain might grab me in its gravita-
tional pull.

Bo is unfazed, peering down calmly at the mountain to
see if he can spot any sign of the crash. I start to realize
that, when he looks out at these mountains, he sees many
crash sites. Bo tells me that, if he's teaching someone to
fly who is cocky and dangerously confident, he gives them
a gruesome ghost tour of the mountains to shock them
into accepting that humility is necessary here, that things
can go wrong. Not far from the spot where Joe crashed,
there's the spot on the Diadems where an American pilot
was killed; here's the area, over the Lindis Ridge, where
a British father and son crashed and died together in a
glider; this is Horrible, where a Japanese man died in the
front seat of a two-seater glider; here's the Omarama
Saddle, where a New Zealand pilot fell to his death.

Bo is resigned to these accidents. 'I know,' he says, 'that
someone else I know will die in a gliding accident in the
future; it will happen again, and it might happen to me.'
He accepts the risk of soaring in the mountains, but
he quickly goes on to point out that, in New Zealand,
fishermen and kayakers regularly drown, base jumpers
often crash. The glaciers surrounding Mount Cook hold
many bodies of mountaineers, trapped and frozen, unable
to decompose and return to the earth properly. People
pursue risky outdoor activities in this landscape; stuff

happens. 'Life without flying . . . Well . . .' he says, trailing off. It's clearly impossible for him to imagine. What's unsaid is that flying is worth dying for.

It is the shadowy side of this exultant sport and it's been kept hidden from me, or rather I've kept it hidden from myself. There is unnecessary death up here in the skies, as well as rapturous life. I am coming to understand that Gavin, Bo, Lemmy, G, Philip, Jenny, Yvonne, Terry and the rest are used to losing people. They are full of sorrow for Joe, but quickly put that to one side in order to fly again.

I can't work out what I feel about this response. What else could they do? Stop flying? And for how long? I don't know what other pilots feel about Joe's death, because I don't feel able to ask. And now a kind of silence has surrounded the subject – it has become taboo. But I know the partners of pilots take on the emotional burden of anxiety. Jenny explains that she and her husband, John, have an agreement that, if she hits her head three times on the canopy in severe turbulence, it's time to come home.

'She's a safe pilot,' John says. 'She tells me she doesn't take unnecessary risks.' He turns to his wife. 'You're always very good at their safety things, aren't you?' he says, reassuring himself.

Jenny nods silently.

*

Over the last few days, and since Joe's death, the life at Omarama and the world of extreme flying that I've become so embedded in has begun to make me feel a little uneasy. So, when Justin and his wife, Gillian, invite me and a group of pilots for dinner at Irishman's Creek, the farm where Dick Georgeson grew up, and where Justin now lives, I find I'm relieved at the chance to get away from the airfield for an evening. Ricco plays his cuatro and sings to us. Gillian shows me her collection of birds' nests, laid out in rows on a table. They are made from tussock grass, merino wool, lichen and moss. I peer intently into the comforting, delicate interior of one, and reach my finger in to gently touch the interwoven wool and twigs. It is good to feel something of birdlife.

During the drive back, in the dark, along the unlit, straight road past Lake Pukaki, the inside of the car glows blue-green from the dash. We are a multinational group from Japan, Austria, China, Canada and the U.K., but the language gap is bridged by song when we all break into 'Supercalifragilisticexpialidocious'. I'm not sure who started it, but everyone knows the words, Hollywood gobbledygook bringing us together. As we speed through the darkness, singing, a series of thuds accompany our music, like a strange bass, and black shapes fly out of the edge of the headlights. Rabbits. They are everywhere. I think of the kahus, which, tomorrow, once the sun has heated up the road enough to create thermals, will circle overhead before descending to feast on our roadkill.

Chapter Thirteen

The Edge

'The control of fear is a necessary part of the inner
work of flight.'

William Langewiesche

Gabriel has a sixth sense in the sky; he is the only pilot I
know who turns the audio vario off. He can register the
lift quicker than the instrument, he says, which is always
a split-second behind him. And the vario can incorrectly
read a gust as a rising thermal. Gabriel, on the other hand,
always knows the difference. He learned to fly gliders in
the French Alps, aged fifteen, and has now been flying for
ten years. When he first started flying, he says, he thought
mechanically, but now he feels the air. And, when he
changed his way of flying, 'The sky felt completely new.'
He recalls how, one day, early on in his flying, he looked
up through a huge mountain-shaped cumulus, thousands
of feet high, and felt like he was at the bottom of a valley,
peering up at a Himalayan giant. The sky is a landscape to
Gabriel.

I'm fortunate to have the opportunity of a flying lesson

with Gabriel, one afternoon in March. It's remarkably quiet without the audio vario, the only sound the rushing of the air over the wings and fuselage, and the cockpit seems to expand. Gabriel releases over the Nursery, finds some ridge and thermal lift, up to the Ewe Range, and then flies out over the Lindis Range. There's a quietness about him as he concentrates on tuning in to the sensations of the air.

I take over to guide us up the Ahuriri Valley, but we begin to get low, so Gabriel takes back control, looking over at Longslip, the nearest land-out strip. He is silent; if we get any lower, we'll have to head over there to land. But, somehow, we crawl up the side of Ben Avon, inching upwards to a few thousand feet above the ridge; I take control and fly out over the Mackenzie Basin, where we've altitude enough to play.

Gabriel demonstrates thermal flying in a way I've not experienced before. He feels his way into some lift and tells me to really tune in to the sensation; he then flies purposefully away from it and finds its edge, and I tune in to that. I take over and want to find the edge of the thermal myself. We are in lift; I fly away from it and find the sink. Gabriel encourages me to explore the lift without relying on the beeping of the audio vario. We sink dramatically; he takes over and flies us back into rising air. He's calm and thoughtful, intensely focused.

He describes the sensations of lift and sink using the analogy of going up and down in a lift. When a lift sets off, he explains, you feel a lurch, the same jolt you get on entering a thermal, but once it is ascending at a regular speed, the sensation dies away. Then, as the lift begins to slow, you feel a sinking feeling, even though it's continuing to go up. Such is the puzzling response of the inner ear, brain and stomach. Gabriel labels these sensations lightness, heaviness and nothing. He has a colour-coding system in his mind to identify the strength of the lightness or heaviness he feels, a kind of imagined synaesthesia for navigating the sky. He visualizes warping bubbles growing and passing away. The thermals around us may be invisible to the eye, but he feels their lift and sink in colour.

Gabriel's technique, based on a decade of intense learning at a crucial age, when the brain is like a sponge, shines a spotlight on the sensations of flying, bringing them out in sharper detail. He describes everything so neatly, so clearly that, for the first time since I've been in New Zealand, I've some clarity about what it might actually be like to fly, to read the sky as a gifted pilot. Without the baffling science and technicalities, this seems pure – it makes sense. I can only just follow him, but slowly, as we fly, I begin to interpret my sensations a little more accurately. And I choose colour codes of my own – purple for heaviness and yellow for lightness. I'm deeper into my flying body.

Gabriel recently spent some time with an indigenous shaman in Peru, undergoing various rites of passage, which he says improved his flying, changing his approach from a sense of controlling and acting, to one of receiving. Now, when he flies, he says, 'I make my mind silent and quiet, and feel where I want to go.' Thinking is slower than his intuitive feel for what's happening to the air, he explains. 'The brain is still there,' he goes on, 'but intuition and intellect work together.'

There's something slightly otherworldly about Gabriel, something of his namesake, but I now see that his intuitive flying skills are informed by a pitch-perfect understanding of the air and an embodied response to it that's entirely rational and clearly thought through. He's using what sports psychologists call the 'implicit system', where he has such a depth of understanding and experience of what he's doing that he can trust his intuitive, implicit mind. He has become a tuning fork in the sky.

I discuss this with Jenny, later, on the ground. 'Some people fly by feel,' she says, 'some fly intellectually, as though the flight is a three-dimensional chess game.' Throughout her body, she says, all her senses are alert, but she uses her hearing in particular, and is highly sensitized to the sound of the glider moving through the air.

Gabriel's approach to extreme flying in the mountains might label him an adventure athlete or 'adrenalin junkie', but this is not about adrenalin at all; in fact, Gabriel considers adrenalin a defensive process.

In one of his morning lectures, Gavin talked about 'adrenalin management', and explained that you don't want to get flooded with adrenalin because your brain and body will go into flight, freeze or fight modes, none of which will help you in the air; there's no grizzly bear coming at you, so playing dead won't help, running isn't possible and there's nothing to fight. The pilot must try to manage the flow of adrenalin to maintain clear thinking. 'If it comes upon you, remain calm and look for options,' he said.

The only thing that adrenalin helps with is slowing down the perception of time, speeding up your thinking and responses. 'Time slows dramatically during major excitements,' says Justin, when I ask him about it. But, other than that, adrenalin just makes you feel sick and shaky. It's of little use to glider pilots.

*

On a cool autumn afternoon in March, a text from Gabriel arrives, asking if I can be ready to fly in five minutes. I put on an adult diaper (there's no time for the silicon Shewee-style contraption), fill my water bottle, slap on some suncream and rush to the launch point.

Gabriel had texted me from the air; he was just coming in to land in the glider Romeo Zulu. He'd been flying into the mountains that morning with a Polish pilot when Gavin radioed. Gavin was 14,000 feet in the wave, heading towards Mount Cook, and asked Gabriel to join him and professional photographer Marty Taylor, to take what they hoped would be some spectacular shots of a glider soaring in the wave. Gavin was flying in Quebec Quebec, his extra-large Duo Discuss, and Marty had attached a high-powered lens on to one of Quebec Quebec's wings, controlled from a laptop he kept on his knee, cramped in the back. This would be an epic flight — less a flying lesson than a wild ride into the mountains.

I do the aerotow well, then Gabriel takes charge, finds some pushy, strong thermals over the Nursery Ridge, and we are soon up at 5,000 feet. We circle and wheel, no beeping audio vario, the air rushing all around us as we spiral upwards and Romeo Zulu creaks like a ship. Hot sun streaks into the canopy, still harsh, even in autumn, and I suddenly feel self-conscious that I'm not wearing deodorant. I rarely wear it, these days, due to scares about chemicals and breast cancer, but in the confined cockpit, steeped in blazing sunshine, I can feel my skin dampening.

But the temperature noticeably cools as we ascend to 6,000, 7,000, 8,000 feet, and I'm glad I remembered to put on my down jacket in the rush. We bank this way and that, and I feel every bump of rising air. The ground shrinks as we get closer to the bottom of the cumulus layer. The dry plain of the Mackenzie Basin looks parched and hungry. I take out the tiny notebook and pencil I keep in my jacket pocket and jot down a few observations.

'You're hunting for words, while I hunt for thermals,' Gabriel sing-songs from behind me, and I laugh. He's right; words have a certain feel to them, too — a lightness or heaviness that I sense in my body, like rising or sinking air.

The sun shatters into multicoloured strands of light through the canopy, and, lower now, at five p.m., casts long autumn shadows that glance across the shrinking land below. We fly up the Lindis Ridge, move into a bowl where Gabriel hopes to find ridge lift, but it isn't working and we lose some height. We move over to Ben Avon, and the air becomes rough with strong thermals and rotor turbulence clashing and mixing.

Gabriel thinks we can make contact with the wave over the other side of Ben Avon, in the lee of the Dingle Ridge. He decides we need to get over the pass here, and so he begins to explore the edge of the ridge lift. The air is unstable, tumbling down and rolling over itself. We fly away from the rough air, but then turn back directly towards it. Gabriel asks if my straps are tight, then he drops the nose. We speed up to eighty knots and head directly into the turbulent air to be bounced over the top of the pass.

Gabriel finds weak, smooth wave, and soon we rise up through the rotor, through a gap in the cumulus layer, so we're level with the clouds and I can see how shredded and torn they are by the turbulence. We climb well above the clouds, speeding upwards on the invisible wave, and the ground disappears. The sky is huge and getting bigger.

We reach 10,000 feet, put on cannulas, start the oxygen flow and then track fast in the direction of Mount Cook, flying over the Huxley Valley, the Hopkins Valley, the Neumann Range and the Dobson Valley. Then, ahead and slightly below, I see Quebec Quebec, flying deeper into the mountains. Its giant white twenty-metre wings are dwarfed by the environment; it looks tiny and vulnerable. We fly together over Mount Sefton and on towards the higher peaks.

In the distance, Mount Cook rises up through the clouds. Flying fast, at seventy knots, we reach it, and the lower clouds part, revealing the glaciers beneath. The mountain has a presence that's neither welcoming nor hostile. One half of it is in complete shadow, the other in bright, low sunlight. It grows enormous as we approach the summit and fly along the jagged top of its peak, at 12,400 feet. Staring out at the mountain that has claimed so many lives, I look down on the grey moraine below, where the Tasman Glacier melts into Lake Tasman. Beyond the peak is a chaotic mass of rock and ice and cloud.

A jagged ridge behind Mount Cook casts a long, crisp shadow on to the white glacier: an open sharp-toothed jaw. My heart thumps like a drum as we fly back over the summit. I peer down into crevasses 10,000 feet below, still distinguishable from up here; they must be big enough to swallow us whole. Gavin comes on the radio and asks Gabriel to fly a couple of loops over the peak. Gabriel drops the nose gently, we speed up, the mountain comes towards us, he pulls back on the stick and we perform what feels like a slow arc in the sky (in truth, we're doing a hundred knots); at the top of the loop, the mountain upside down, we seem to hang in space, the rush of air silenced momentarily, before we speed down the other side of the circle. The G-force presses into me as my body trebles in weight. Towards the end of the loop, Gabriel puts the glider into a small bunt and my legs lift off in the negative G. The movement from positive to negative G is like a strange see-saw inside the body.

We soar over the Tasman and Hooker Glaciers that surround Mount Cook, and head back along the ridge again. The cumulus layer beneath us reaches out to where the oceans begin on either side of the island, and, from 14,000 feet, in the crystal-clear air, I can see both coasts – the Tasman Sea to the west, the South Pacific to the east. I find myself staring fixedly at the distant coastline, and it is in the moment that I feel the urge to turn away from the mountain and look towards the sea that I know something is wrong. I've never flown so close to such a monster as Mount Cook. I feel like a fly on the back of a giant animal that might flick me away with its tail at any moment.

We fly just above the mountain, which seems to grow larger, to morph and become more imposing as the flight continues, like a face slowly changing expression from benign to sinister. The Tasman Glacier sliding down the mountain and around its base begins to look like a swollen, monstrous serpent.

We fly on towards the north side of Mount Cook and suddenly, without any warning, we're tumbling down a black hole of sinking rotor. I scream, grab my straps and hang on to them with both hands, the only movement I can make, ineffectual though it is. Blackness envelops my mind as we continue to be thrown around above glacial crevasses and rocks, and I feel like we're falling down into an abyss. I close my eyes, breathe the bottled oxygen, but it's too late – adrenalin has me in its grip. My thighs shake and I know I'm beginning to panic. 'Get us out of here,' I tell Gabriel, who is quiet in the back.

This wave is deceptive. The lift is silky smooth, but, at its edge and beneath it, the rotor can be tremendous, can break up an airframe. It's like a soft cat's paw that suddenly unleashes its claws. It is all I can do not to grab the handle and open the canopy to bail out with my parachute into the crevasses below. It feels as though the air is aggressively attacking us, as though violence has broken out. The dark, clear truth that the elements don't care about us in our little glass-fibre engineless bird hits me full in the face. It's a cold universe all of a sudden, and I am overcome with helplessness. I feel trapped, buried alive in the sky.

Gabriel gets on the radio and tells Gavin it's too rough here, we need to get away from the rotor. Gabriel warns me that we have to fly back through that rough air to get to the smoother lift on the other side. I grip my straps and we head into it again; our wings bend, we thump up and down, the air roars, and then it's over and we're out.

I bite my tongue as Gavin comes on the radio and asks Gabriel to fly again along the ridge of Mount Cook. Having got this far, he and Marty want to make the most of this opportunity to get shots of a tiny glider amid the rocks and ice. Gabriel tells Gavin that I'm not doing well, Gavin says OK, understood, but we agree to continue. Gabriel pulls the air brakes to make us descend a third of the way down Mount Cook. It now looms above us as we soar alongside the rocks; the crevasses look as though they've been slashed open by claws. It feels as if we're inside the mountain, in the guts of the rocks. My heart pumps fast, and it's only the oxygen puffing up my nose that reminds me I'm still breathing. Above us, most of the sky is shut out by rock and ice.

I can't see Gabriel's face, so I have no idea what he is thinking or feeling, but there's tension in his voice. I don't know if this is because we're in danger and he's flying on the outer limit of his skills, or because he's concerned about me. Whichever it is, he offers no words of reassurance. Gabriel is a brilliant pilot and I'm as safe as anyone can be in this situation, which in truth is not entirely safe. This is the extreme edge of glider flying and it's my edge too; I have finally found it: I can experience total all-consuming fear.

Ideas about where the limits lie – my psychological limits, the limitations of this aircraft and Gabriel's flying skills – all swirl about inside my adrenalin-darkened mind as I try to distinguish between perceived and actual risk. I keep quiet as we continue to fly lower in the mountains, getting closer to where I know the rotor will be, rolling and tumbling below. We could hit it at any moment.

By the time we rise up in the wave and ridge lift and fly yet again over the summit of Mount Cook, I am desperately frightened at the thought of more turbulence. It's early evening; the sun is low, shining on the Tasman Sea out west, which is smooth beaten silver. We fly away from the peak, towards Mount Sefton, and into more rough air. The rotor is horrendous and, as we buck and the wings bow, I finally crack and tell Gabriel that I can't do this any longer – I need to get down now.

I have managed to keep going for an hour or so after the tremendous rotor to the north of Mount Cook, but I can no longer cope with my emotions. I'm failing miserably at Gavin's 'adrenalin management'. Odd images and memories come to mind: a glass of cool water placed on a bare table; lying on my back on a flat, newly mown lawn; deep-sea diving. All I can think of is getting back to the ground, which has never looked so appealing. I want to get down, away, out. For the first time in eleven months, since I started free flying, I'm truly afraid. I look down at the flat braided river valley, where the glacial melt flows into the lake, and long for the land.

Gavin heads off into the rotor, towards Mount Sefton, and Gabriel turns to fly along the Ben Ohau Range, on the edge of Lake Pukaki, where there might be some smooth wave intact. The nearest land-out site is Mount Cook airfield, on the edge of the lake, but the wind is too strong to land. The closest safe landing area is Twizel airfield, so we radio ahead to ask a tow pilot to fly out to meet us there, so Gabriel can be relaunched to fly back to Omarama.

This flight has sent me to a place in myself that's sharp, craggy and rough, difficult to navigate and impossible to control. Gabriel and I are both looking inward – me, at the raging storm inside my brain and body; Gabriel, at the sensations of lift as he navigates the collapsing wave along the Ben Ohau Range. Keeping my gaze focused straight ahead, I concentrate on breathing and, as soon as I spot the airfield, I start to feel better. It's just twenty minutes away. Hold on, I think. No screaming, no passing out, no trying to leap out of the cockpit.

We descend fast through the rotor, and the airstrip

rushes beneath us. We land and come to a stop, and I tear the cannula from my face and grapple with my straps to struggle out of the glider. I feel stupid for asking Gabriel to land, and sorry that I screamed and didn't seem to trust him, but I am exhausted from the flight, from the calm awe and the terror and the panic. Gabriel climbs out behind me and gives me a hug.

Not long after, the towplane arrives. Ash Hurndell, the pilot, attaches a rope to the front of the glider, I run the wing, Gabriel takes off, and I am left alone on the airstrip, the light fading fast, waiting for Bo to pick me up in his car. I can see the mountains in the distance, thankfully small again, now a harmless, flat, black silhouette. I've no doubt that Gavin and Gabriel will make it back to Omarama safely. I scuff my feet in the dust and dry grass.

I'm curious about fear. It is powerful, but delicate, has lace-like intricacies, is visual and sensual. For me, fear is a falling feeling inside the guts, tunnel vision, and blackness in the brain. I can deal with fear — I have to; I have faced, and will face for the rest of my life, regular check-ups where doctors search inside my body for things that might be killing me. I cope, I get through. In some ways, I am sure my illness built my capacity to face fear, but in other ways it made me more vulnerable, because now I know things won't necessarily be all right. If you've experienced an earthquake, you know that the ground can shift suddenly beneath your feet. I know that things can go wrong in an instant and lives can be changed forever. It might not all end well. Trying to get some hold on fear is like circling over a mountain; it shape-shifts as you move, showing dramatically different sides from different points of view.

Perhaps I have been using free flying to build my resilience, to cope with what I face back on the earth. I wonder if I have become addicted to flying in order to get to know fear and risk better. But now, standing abandoned on an airstrip, I know that, in that flight with Gabriel, I went too far. My amygdala, the almond-shaped section of the brain that registers fear, erupted, flooding me with unmanageable amounts of adrenalin. I have found that part of me that will kick back against risk, draw a line in what I can endure. The experience was intimate and real. Thrown around at 11,000 feet with no real skills of my own that might save my life, the quaking of my body was an understandable response. It means I am alive.

Gavin told me, months ago, that he liked to encourage people to press up against their 'personal envelope', and I know I have now; in fact, I've fallen through the edge of it. I thought I was beyond fear, wanted to remain beyond it, but now I think I can reluctantly admit to myself that there's something very honest, very human about coming back to fear.

I pace the airfield in the silence and growing darkness, until I see the headlights of Bo's thirty-year-old Mitsubishi turn off the main road and come towards me. He's waving at me through the windshield, grinning. Bo assumes I have asked Gabriel to land at Twizel so that he can pick me up for our appointment at the Mount John Observatory, an astronomy research base for the University of Canterbury that offers night-sky tours and the opportunity to gaze through their telescopes. I don't disillusion him of this idea at first; I need just a little longer to recover from the flight. Lemmy, Trevor and Martin, an Austrian instructor, are squeezed into the back of the car, so I haul myself into the front seat and we speed off, throwing up gravel as we join the main road to Tekapo.

The electric lights of Tekapo town are kept low to prevent light pollution interfering with the research taking place at the top of Mount John, where scientists peer out of the darkness each night, into the southern sky. The shop windows are softly lit and the street lights capped to project downwards what low light they shine. The whole town has an eerie, secretive feel. It reminds me a little of home, where the nights are dark and close in.

On the farm in Wales, on cloudy or moonless nights, there's no difference between having your eyes open or closed, and since leaving the place where I grew up, I have often felt over-lit, have craved darkness. The Brecon Beacons National Park is a dark-skies area and a draw for British astronomers hoping for cloudless skies to access the heavens. I can tell what time of year it is and what time of night by the passage of some constellations, particularly the Plough and Orion's Belt as their position shifts over the barn roof at home and through the branches of the old walnut tree on the edge of the yard, against the curve of the hill on the opposite side of the valley.

We leave the car and hop on an observatory bus, driven without headlights by a trained driver up the winding road of Mount John. We are met by our night-sky guide and led along unlit footpaths. I sneak into a bathroom we pass, hoping to get out of the unused diaper I am still wearing, but I fear losing the group in the dark, so I change my mind and run out to catch up with them. I'll just have to keep it on.

Our guide points to various constellations with a laser and we see the glittering Milky Way and the Southern Cross. We watch the moon rise, through a telescope, the features of its upside-down face in perfect detail. We take turns to peer through telescopes at the Wishing Well star cluster, which looks like a dish of sparkling diamonds. I bend down and press my eye to a scope and see Saturn, shimmering like a spinning silver coin inside its rings.

I shuffle in my nappy, my bottom feels large and round, though nobody can see it in the dark; we can't even see each other's faces. I have moved rapidly from terror and turbulence above the mountains, to standing on one, peering at the outer solar system and at new stars forming outside our galaxy, in the Tarantula Nebula of the Magellanic Clouds. The shift in scale is vast. The day sky had terrified me, and now I am looking through the night sky, through the invisible atmosphere in which all that happened, to the stars beyond.

*

The following day, I head to the terminal building to find Gavin. I am determined that he and Gabriel should reassure me that I had nothing to fear yesterday. I want to teach myself that lesson, to conquer my new-found terror. I find him in the office and corner him.

'Wave has a rough edge,' Gavin says, 'and sometimes it's not clear where the edge is until you bump up against it.' He continues, with a twinkle in his eye, 'But I would have ignored you, when you said you wanted to land, and flown on through the rotor, back to Omarama, and just let you scream.'

We walk over to the Kahu for coffee with Gabriel. I ask Gabriel if I had been safe yesterday.

'No,' he says. 'Don't go gliding if you want to be safe.'

There is no attempt to smooth over the experience or placate me. My request for reassurance has been met with sangfroid. I receive no sympathy and certainly no empathy. These pilots are so experienced that they can't identify with my need for reassurance. I'm suddenly aware of how far away I am from this mentality; it seems like madness to me, wilful disregard for a very natural instinct to keep myself safe. It's as though, suddenly, a great chasm has opened up – Gavin and Gabriel on one side of it, and me on the other.

Bo warned me that a pilot needs to build up to this kind of flight, that it would be scary, demanding, that I should take care not to push myself too much. I had not taken heed. And now I am annoyed, anxious that the pilots here might see me as fearful. Many of them don't know what I've endured over the previous few years, how courageously I have faced the disintegration of my life and body. I want to stand on a table in the Kahu and shout, 'I am not weak. I am strong. I am not afraid.'

What I find disconcerting is that there is no room for my fear at Omarama. I can't find anyone to talk to about this experience who has any real sympathy; Lemmy dismisses it, even Bo agrees with what Gabriel said. If the only way I can fly is while I am convinced I am safe, then I shouldn't be flying at all.

I begin to wonder if perhaps my fear, this new, violent emotion, is being rejected by the pilots as a means of continuing to deny their own — what little they have left, after so many years of flying in these mountains. Few pilots, especially men, are willing to acknowledge that they ever feel afraid. But I know that fear erupts in their dreams. Gavin, G and Bo all have dreams about searching for somewhere to land, only to find, over and over, that there are power lines everywhere.

One evening, a few weeks ago, G told me about a dream he had: 'I was flying down the road, at low level. I had to stay right in the middle of the road so I didn't hit the glider wings on the fences, but I also had to stay underneath the power lines. Every time I thought I might be able to pull up and climb away, there was another wire in front of me.'

He had another vivid dream where he was flying amongst huge trees: 'Really big, a bit like a bird flying through ordinary-sized trees; I was trying to weave in and out of them without hitting anything.'

G is also haunted by real flying incidents. 'I have a

recurring nightmare,' he said, 'where something appalling has happened, but I can't get a message out on the telephone. It won't dial correctly. Those dreams began after watching a glider crash from very close up – both pilots died – and I was the one who ran for the phone. And fumbled it, of course.'

The women pilots are much more open in talking about their fear. 'I definitely get scared,' admits Jenny. 'My muscles clench, I get a knot in the stomach.' The paint is wearing thin in the kneeholes of her glider because she tenses her thighs and her knees rise up to press against the bodywork. 'I really don't like being properly frightened,' she says, 'but a little bit of fear adds to the experience. That's partly why we do it. We do it because there is a little bit of risk.' And, she says, 'A little bit of fear keeps you safe . . . If you barrel in, something is more likely to bite you.'

*

It is early April, a couple of days before I am due to fly back to Wales, and I have borrowed a car to drive the sixty miles from Omarama to Mount Cook Village, at the base of the mountain. From the ground, as I drive along its edge, Lake Pukaki seems as big as a sea. I stop the car to look up at Mount Cook's huge triangle of rock and ice, but I can't find the same mountain as the one I flew over.

I drive along the gravel road from Mount Cook Village to Lake Tasman, the old automatic sliding on the gravel as

I brake. I hike up the path to the edge of the lake, admiring the delicate gauze nursery web spider encasements, full of spiderlings, spun on thorn bushes along the way.

A blush of rust-coloured algae clings to the grey rocks on either side of my feet, and tiny white flowers grow in between the cracks. I have no idea what either are called. In looking for the names, here, I know I'm going to run into knotty controversies about whether these are native plants or invasive intruders, choices about their Maori or European names, scientific or colloquial. Crouching to look down at the white flower, gently touching its stem and petals, I'm allowed a brief release from the human controversies in which the plant is no doubt embedded. Naming a thing is different from knowing it.

The frozen river flowing in slow motion down the mountainside into Lake Tasman is a strange, prehistoric sight from the ground. The wall of ice where the glacier ends is covered in grey rock scree, looking dirty compared to the gleaming blue-white ice further up. Icebergs the size of container ships float in the lake. Mount Cook looks benign from here, too, and I understand now how profoundly the mountain is transformed by the weather that surrounds it. A mountain is more than rock rearing up from the ground, I think; it's the sum of the relationship between that rock and the sky it reaches up into and shapes. In a sense, the air around a mountain is an expression of it.

*

I've reached the end of the flying season in New Zealand. Pilots are leaving, like migrating birds, heading for mountain ranges across the world, to teach soaring in the northern hemisphere, in the Sierra Nevadas, the Rockies, the European Alps.

On the morning of the day I am due to leave, I join Gavin in one of the towplanes, sitting next to him on the tiny fold-down seat as we pull someone into the sky. The towplane is a flying tractor, he says, which is a good description of the old agricultural crop sprayer, a GA200. I haven't flown in a glider with Gavin – he's so much in demand during this busy season – but at least now I get the opportunity to spend a little time up in the sky with him.

After the glider has released from us, we head off for a short local flight and wheel around above Mount Horrible, where Gavin's father crashed in a glider, half a century ago. As we come in to land, I look down for the last time at the mile-long grass airstrip and the shiny metal hangars, at the rows of poplars and groups of willow trees. I've been here for only four months, but the time-dilation effect of free flight has made it seem much longer.

'You go away for a long time', wrote travel writer, Paul Theroux, 'and return a different person – you never come all the way back.'

I picture my lost earring somewhere at the bottom of the Ahuriri River, slowly washing downstream in the clear, blue, icy water among the pebbles, little pieces of the mountain that have worn away.

Part Three

The Black Mountains, Wales
&
The Annapurna Range in
the Himalayas, Nepal

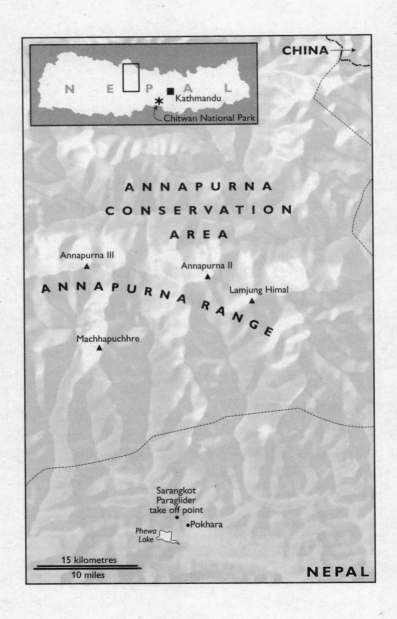

CHINA →

N E P A L

■ Kathmandu

✳
⌐ Chitwan National Park

A N N A P U R N A

C O N S E R V A T I O N

A R E A

Annapurna III
▲

Annapurna II
▲

Lamjung Himal
▲

A N N A P U R N A   R A N G E

Machhapuchhre
▲

Sarangkot
Paraglider
take off point
●
●Pokhara

Phewa
Lake

15 kilometres

10 miles

N E P A L

Chapter Fourteen

Bird Guides

'My heart in hiding
Stirred for a bird'

Gerard Manley Hopkins,
'The Windhover'

I return from New Zealand to spring in the Black Mountains of Wales. On the farm, the lambs are already several weeks old and pronking at dusk, at the top of the field, next to the orchard, throwing themselves into the air. It is strange to have hopped over winter once again, to have returned just as the daffodils are waning. And because I haven't endured those long, cold months when the sun disappears behind the hill opposite the farmhouse by four o'clock, I am not loaded with the normal yearning for spring, which precedes its arrival. The primroses and wood anemones have already emerged in the banks and hedgerows, and where, from early April onwards, I'd usually be looking for the first swallows, checking the diary in which Mum keeps a record of the dates of their arrival in previous years, those little birds are already home again.

The familiar world of the farm has been the bedrock beneath the twisting river of my life, but when I get back, I decide it is time for some space of my own. I have found a simple converted chapel a few miles down the road that I can rent by the month. It is perfect. It demands no commitment, so I can remain light on my feet, able to set off at any moment. I am like a hare, poised and watchful in its temporary form.

My chapel has four large arched windows that suck in the sun, and the single main room feels like a lung inflated with light. Pen y Fan is visible from the west-facing window. At night, upstairs in the bedroom, I can hear scrabbling sounds coming from inside the wall. Birds, I'm not sure what kind, are nesting in the crack near where I lay my head. The chicks hiss and chirp at night and when the adults return to feed them, so it sounds as though the stone wall of the chapel is alive.

There is a window close and level to the head of the bed, and every night I sleep with it wide open. One dawn, as I surface from sleep, I hear the bubbling sound of a small stream nearby, until thought creeps in and I remember where I am, that there is no stream. My dream brain has turned the dawn chorus into a river of birdsong; I see it flowing past in my mind's eye as I fall back into a doze with the delicious sensation of floating on a stream of song.

A few days later, on a warm spring morning when the

herb Robert is in full cirrus swing in the hedgerows, Polly and Nick, my hiking friends, visit the chapel and we walk to the farm, arriving from the hill above it rather than the road. Now I have stitched the chapel to the farm, joining them together with the thread of my footsteps.

*

It is my first flight, back in the U.K., and Bo and I are soaring above the airfield. From the moment I returned, I have been keen to see again the delicate beauty of this place from above, these soft familiar hills. From the air, the landscape looks bridal at this time of year, covered in spring blossom, cow parsley lining each field and lane. And yet, despite the beauty, and the warm recognition that home brings, I am finding it hard to feel my way into flying again. It is as though my fear, after that flight with Gabriel, has hardened me up, stiffened me, made me less liquid, less adaptable. I had trusted my time in the sky until that flight, trusted Bo implicitly, but having been flung around by the sky in New Zealand, there is some residual anxiety. The old wooden K13 feels flimsy after the glass and carbon-fibre Duo Discuses we flew in Omarama, but I also feel more intimate with the sky here, which howls into the cockpit through gaps where the canopy meets the fuselage. The spring sky over the Black Mountains is far less boisterous than the sky over the Southern Alps – cumulus clouds are small and bouncy, the air full of birds and the moisture of a damp April. Up ahead, we can see curtains of rainclouds floating over Hay-on-Wye and the Wye River; they create rainbows close to the ground, far below us.

Over the next few days, I find myself rushing between the chapel and the gliding club, but after just a few flights, the weather stops all flying. It is too windy, too wet — one of the wettest springs on record. The rain falls and falls, the river bursts its banks, fledglings drown in sodden nests and sheep limp across fields with foot rot from the waterlogged earth. The land is drenched, running, turning to liquid as though the very sky is falling, and there is no flying for weeks. Bo is outraged, pacing the deserted, muddy airfield in waterproof jacket and wellington boots in frustrated desperation. The sky is his habitat and he has been banished. The psychological impact is immense. We are all grounded.

But, for me, this rained-off spring has created a pause in my flying at just the right time. Things have changed and, now I am being forced back to the ground, I begin to sense a new phase in the process in which I am immersed. Since returning from New Zealand, my flights have become edged with an awareness of the dangers of this sport. I can no longer believe that gliding is risk-free, because I know — have seen and felt — that it is not. I now understand much better the skills required to soar without an engine safely and effectively, and I am in awe of them. Now, I realize I would have to give myself, all my time and all my money to it in order to become an even moderately good pilot, and I'm not sure that's what I want. I don't want to feel like those pilots whose time on solid land is only ever a wished-away waiting period before leaping upwards again. I want to be able to live on the ground. I want to be able to love the sky from down here.

I spend time in the chapel reading my flying notebooks, poring over the things I have seen and learned and felt in the sky. And what comes up again and again is birds. The times I've flown close to soaring birds, as well as with swifts and swallows, have burnt into my memory. They are charged experiences, full of something I can't quite grasp.

There is a particular fascination and thrill in soaring with birds, especially raptors, because they fly in the same way as a glider, following essentially the same aeronautical principles. But I had no bird encounters in New Zealand, and I realize now how much I missed flying with them. Though Gavin told me that he once came across a solitary cormorant at 9,000 feet, and a black-backed gull at 10,000 feet, near Mount Cook, those were unusual sightings in New Zealand. If the buzzards and kites disappeared from the Welsh skies, I would feel bereft, as if a deep part of my flying experience had been ripped away.

The Black Mountains and Brecon Beacons are an ideal flying site for two other forms of free flight: hang-gliding and paragliding, and paragliders can be seen here most weekends, circling low in thermals or surfing along the ridges. During these rain-soaked days at the gliding club, I realize that many of the members are paragliders and hang-gliders too, and every one of these pilots tells of encounters with birds that have dug into their memories, like a raptor's claws. The lives of free-flight pilots are thick with these mysterious moments, and, over the next few weeks, their stories become a flock of images murmurating in my mind, shape-shifting as different themes emerge.

I have heard countless stories about birds acting as guides, showing pilots the way to invisible rising air, from swallows marking the convergence line above a ridge in Lasham, where Justin Wills once flew, to Gabriel following vultures in the Pyrenees and having to trust they were descending only because they knew there was strong lift in the distance. But the tales of bird encounters that seem driven deepest into pilots' memories are the ones when birds have saved them.

The story that sits in my mind, as I go over my notes in the chapel one evening, is John Silvester's. John is a one-time British paragliding champion and distance-record holder, who got into difficulty when he flew an unexplored route in the Karakorum Range of the Himalayas, in Pakistan. Flying over a glacier, John was separated from Eddie, his fellow pilot. He lost altitude and lift, and was forced to crawl above the glacier, staring down into its crevasses. He knew he would be doomed if he landed. After struggling for two hours on the edge of catastrophe, hypoxic at 22,000 feet, without oxygen, he was concentrating on staying aloft in every scrap of lift, when he looked up and saw what he thought was a high-flying jet overhead. As he stared, it suddenly banked to turn and John realized it was a falcon, its silver-white wings catching the light reflected off the ice below. He was no longer alone. John was able to follow the path the bird mapped in the sky above him and he eventually made it to safety. Twenty-four hours later, and reunited with Eddie, the two men sat down to dissect their flight. John was convinced that his white-winged bird must have been a gyrfalcon, but that wasn't possible: gyrfalcons are Arctic raptors – they have never been seen in the Himalayas. And there are no other white falcons that John could possibly have seen at 22,000 feet.

I wonder if perhaps, exhausted and under immense stress, John hallucinated the soaring raptor in a version of the 'third man syndrome', whereby people in life-threatening situations perceive a benign presence who seems to be there to help or to offer support. Shackleton was the first to admit to this experience during his expedition to the South Pole, and Charles Lindbergh, on his epic solo transatlantic flight, in 1926, was joined by a host of 'magical travelling companions', as Jung called them. John recognizes the possibility that he hallucinated the bird, and the experience remains a mystery to him, but, either way, John's falcon saved his life – for a brief moment, he was entirely dependent on a wild animal.

But pilots must also exercise judgement, a local falconer and paraglider pilot, Martin Cray, tells me. He was saved on a tandem paragliding flight in Texas by a soaring hawk. He and a friend were going for a distance-record attempt, across the state, on a boiling-hot summer day in June. They were in the middle of nowhere when they got very low. To land in forty-degree heat would have been extremely dangerous, but Martin suddenly spotted something in the distance, and he was sure it was a red-tailed hawk, soaring up ahead. The red-tailed hawk is a big, stocky kind of buzzard, whose weight means it needs thermals to fly. It was vital that Martin correctly identify the bird. The paraglider would have to descend towards it and, if Martin was wrong, if it turned out to be a lighter Harris hawk, they'd be on the ground in the heat, fifty kilometres from roads and help. Luckily, Martin was right, and soon the two men and the bird were ascending.

It's not just size that you need to keep in mind when choosing to follow birds in flight. 'Stork groups, for example,' explains Benjamin Bachmeier, a German glider pilot, 'are disciplined when it comes to thermalling, the whole group circling neatly on the same trajectory behind a lead bird. That makes it very easy to fly with them and they don't seem to mind at all.' Buzzards are the complete opposite; they also sometimes fly in groups in thermals, but a buzzard thermal is much more difficult to join than a stork thermal; it's messy and they circle in no order or consistent direction, which means that collisions are a risk.

There are many stories about difficult encounters with eagles, in particular. Territorial and solitary hunters, eagles can regard gliders or paragliders as competition, especially during breeding season, and they have been known to attack, often to the detriment of the poor eagle. Benjamin says that he has goosebumps every time he encounters a golden eagle in the Alps, after a recent trip to Austria.

Rising on lift up the side of a ridge, he arrived at the top to see a pair of nesting eagles. They launched at the glider, flying in front of him to stall in mid-air, before turning their bodies into bullet shapes, readying for attack. Benjamin dropped out of the thermal and escaped, but he came close to collision.

Paragliding close to a steppe eagle in Nepal, Martin remembers receiving a warning display, the bird dropping its huge claws as it passed him, reminding him that it could tear a flimsy wing. Martin found himself audibly apologizing to the eagle as he dropped away to give it some space.

Talking to each of these pilots, hearing their stories, it becomes clear that attitudes to birds on the ground don't apply in the sky. On the ground, it may be the eagle we revere – a symbol of empire, strength, importance – but it is the more traditionally reviled bird, the vulture, that most free-flight pilots love.

Some species of vulture are among the largest soaring birds alive today, and they, together with the albatross, are the birds that fly most like a glider, their heavy bodies relying on natural lift in the sky to keep them aloft. Unlike eagles, vultures are communal flying birds, used to soaring together in groups, relying on each other to find carrion, so flying with them is easy – they simply accept your presence.

Enjoyable tales of soaring with vultures abound. In Omarama, Jenny Wilkinson told me how she flew with vultures in Spain, circling in a thermal surrounded by a dozen of them, their three-metre wingspans reaching out

towards her own wings. She recalled with utter amaze-
ment making full eye-contact with them: 'You knew they
were looking at you,' she said. 'It was amazing to share the
sky with something else that's flying and climbing in the
same way as you are.'

Although many free-flight pilots use soaring birds as lift
markers, it might work the other way too. 'They come to
you,' says John Silvester, of the vultures he encountered
in the Himalayas. 'They come to take a look at you.' He's
watched them preening in the air on the wing next to him,
picking ticks off themselves and eating them.

'Vultures,' says Benjamin Bachmeier, are the most
'uncomplicated creatures to fly with.' He encounters
them in Europe, mostly in the Pyrenees and the southern
part of the Alps, where he flies with bearded, Egyptian,
cinereous and griffon vultures. Successful extended reintroduction programmes have massively increased the
numbers of vultures in these mountains in the last few
years. 'They are peaceful, calm flyers,' Benjamin says, 'and
they naturally follow the same thermal routes through the
mountains as glider pilots do.'

He describes a complex route through the heart of the
Écrins Mountains, the southernmost peaks of the Alps, a
'maze of rocks which is only accessible if you are in the
right place at the right time.' A vulture rose up from a
ridge below and flew close to Benjamin's glider, they
ascended and circled together to get high, away from the
rocks, and then the bird flew back towards him. It's an
experience that looms large in Benjamin's flying memory;

he had never before been that close to something 'so big, so beautiful and so vulnerable.'

*

I am yearning for the curious experience of sharing the air with a soaring bird once again, mimicking its way of flying. I have missed the strange feeling of entering the realm of another creature, where it is master and I am an imposter; I have missed the unknowability of what that encounter means, I have missed catching a bird's eye and trying to read that look, of warning or of welcome.

One day, in mid-May, when neither Bo nor I have been into the sky for weeks, I am talking to Martin in the briefing room when he tells me about an innovative conservation project in Nepal, run by a Briton called Scott Mason. Scott is a paraglider, and has taught rescued vultures to fly with him. Fascinated, I call Scott the next morning and we discuss our different experiences over a crackly phone line. By the time I hang up, my next move is obvious and I start making arrangements to visit Scott in the foothills of the Himalayas.

Chapter Fifteen

Reimagining Vultures

Pokhara is the second largest town in Nepal, after the capital, Kathmandu, and though this is by no means a pristine environment, it is beautiful. Old cows wander the streets chewing on cardboard boxes, women walk past in colourful floral fabrics, the huge baskets on their backs weighing on the straps across their foreheads, and the air is full of birds. Twenty-five kilometres north of Pokhara and looming over the town is Machhapuchhre, known in English as Fishtail Mountain. It is 23,000 feet high and straddles the boundary of the Annapurna Sanctuary at the end of the Annapurna Range of the Himalayas. Sacred to the god Shiva, and off-limits to climbers, it has never been summited. Behind this sacred mountain rears the Annapurna Range, reaching far up into the sky. The sight of these extraordinary mountains forces your head back. Where I expect to see clouds, I see icy crags in the far distance. My teeth shiver as though I'm biting down on cold rock.

A mile or so outside town, and on the edge of a lake, is Scott's raptor rescue centre, and, next to it, the landing strip for paragliders who fly in and around Pokhara. As soon as I arrive, Scott shows me where I'll be staying – a small, round, straw-roofed hut, from where I can hear the birds shuffling in the aviary next door – and then we walk down to the lake together. From the shore, I look up at a gaggle of multicoloured eyebrows circling in the sky, all following the same direction. They remind me of a child's mobile, or the intricate workings of a clock. The paragliders' risers are invisible, so the black dots of the pilots beneath the wings look as though they are suspended by some impossible force. I can hardly wait to get up there myself.

*

The human imagination has evolved in a world full of birds, and the intertwining of the imagination with vultures seems to go back particularly far. The oldest musical instrument ever found is a flute made of the hollow bone from the wing of a griffon vulture, discovered in the Hohle Fels cave, in Germany, in 2008. This flute is 40,000 years old, made at a time when griffon vultures were common in Europe. The social bonds created through making music are thought to be key to the success of *Homo sapiens* over other hominids, and it is a pleasing thought that our first attempts to create music beyond our voices were with the aid of a flying wing. I imagine an Ice Age human blowing through the bone to create a melody that flew, taking her imagination up into the sky from which the vulture came.

Images of vultures have been found carved on to the

side of the earliest temple ever discovered, at Göbekli Tepe, in south-eastern Turkey – a Neolithic site, approximately 9,000 years old – and vulture artefacts were also found in one of the oldest towns to be unearthed, Çatal Hüyük, also in Turkey, where vulture skulls are embedded in the decorative walls. At Çatal Hüyük, there is also a wall painting that shows a vulture pecking at a headless human form, its legs dismembered.

Perhaps there's no more intimate relationship with a bird than the one humanity has with the vulture, because of this death ritual. Exposure of the human dead to vultures is an ancient practice. The Zoroastrian Parsi community, who originated in ancient Iran, arrived in India in the eighteenth century, and brought their ancient burial traditions with them. These involved placing the dead inside enormous stone 'towers of silence', where the bodies were laid out for vultures to feed on. There are remains of these towers in the deserts of Iran, and, in Mumbai and parts of Gujarat, the practice continues to this day.

Sky burial also still takes place on the high Tibetan plateau in the Himalayas. The frozen earth and lack of wood mean that earth burial and cremation are impractical. Instead, bodies are cut into parts and placed in specific sacred sites in the open for the vultures to consume, thereby carrying the spirit aloft. The vulture is a holy creature to the Tibetans, and this practice continues despite Chinese efforts to suppress it.

It seems that the human fascination with birds exists

somewhere between imagination and zoology, and it can be difficult to distinguish real birds from those flying in the birdscape of our cultural imaginations. This is especially true of the vulture. In Tibet, the vulture may be a holy creature, but in more recent times, in the west, vultures are abhorred – associated with scavenging and treated as omens of death and beneficiaries of battlefields. Where other birds offer metaphors for spirit and soul and freedom, the vulture is simply ugly, base. Death is so hidden in Western culture, and vultures confront us with the truth: with our mortality, our edibility. Culturally, we have such a negative view of these raptors that it influences conservation efforts. Some vulture conservation projects have tackled this head-on and renamed the birds they're trying to save. Since the beginnings of a project to reintroduce them into the wild, the North American turkey vulture has been renamed the Californian condor, and, similarly, the European vulture known as the Lammergeier ('lamb vulture') is now the bearded vulture. Saving these birds is an exercise in rebranding.

*

As we talk, that afternoon, Scott explains that Asia's vultures, too, are under threat. South Asia's vultures and local farmers have long had an extraordinary co-dependency. Many farming families keep a cow, and for years vultures have survived on the carcasses of cows left out for them, relying on the Hinduism that prevents the farmers from eating the cows. But, in the late 1990s, vultures started dying in their millions. Dead cows were dragged out into the countryside and left for the birds, but the vultures were no longer appearing in sufficient numbers to do the important work of cleaning up the dead. Cows would normally be picked clean within twenty-four hours, but the carcasses were now left to rot. Covered in flies and attracting rabid dogs, they threatened to poison water and spread disease.

Scientists worked desperately to find out what it was that was killing the vultures, and, in 2003, it was discovered that diclofenac, an anti-inflammatory drug given to ageing cows, was causing the problem. Part of the reason that vultures are so important in the ecology of Asia is because of the remarkable powers of their stomachs. Full of an extraordinarily strong acid, they have the capacity to clean the meat they consume of all pathogens, including anthrax and botulism. Vultures dispose of carcasses quickly and efficiently, breaking them down so that they can be returned to the earth as fertilizer. But the one thing that vultures' systems cannot process, it was discovered, is diclofenac. By the time the culprit was identified, forty-four million vultures had died, the Oriental white-backed vulture had declined by 99.9 per cent and two other species of vulture, the long-billed and slender-billed, had declined by 97 per cent.

Since the collapse in vulture numbers, the Parsi burial tradition is under threat. Black kites have taken the place of vultures at the towers of silence, but they aren't sufficiently thorough scavengers. The decline in vulture numbers also means that farmers are beginning to have to pay to have carcasses burnt or removed, and hide and bone collectors, who rely on clean carcasses, are struggling to make a living. Nobody realized how tightly this circle of interdependence was woven.

The conservation effort to save Asia's vultures has been multi-pronged. In 2006, diclofenac was banned for veterinary use, and there have been major efforts to remove the drug from circulation. Vulture-breeding programmes have been established, with vultures kept in captivity to safeguard them from extinction, and 'vulture safe zones' are being developed – areas close to vulture colonies, where diclofenac-free carcasses can be put out for them. These are known as 'vulture restaurants'.

*

Scott is dynamic, tenacious and passionate about birds of prey and their conservation in the wild, and it's clear that his primary fascination is with the birds rather than flight. Unlike many pilots, he never dreamed of flying: 'I never longed to be in the air, but looking up at birds flying above me wasn't enough.' He recalls that, during his first tandem flight, on a trip to Nepal in 2001, he saw wild birds soaring close by and realized that paragliding 'provided me with an opportunity to be a part of their world in the sky, to see what they see and do what they do. It was a revelation.' He wondered about the possibility of flying with a trained bird, and then, a while later, was presented with two rescued black-kite chicks.

What started as an experiment soon turned into an obsession for Scott, and, over the coming years, more birds were rescued. Another black kite, Brad, was rescued after being kept in a small cage. He couldn't stretch his wings and had developed a slight deformity as a result. Scott knew that there was no way this bird could survive in the wild, but he successfully trained Brad to fly with him. Despite his wing deformity, Brad was incredibly fast and agile. 'Keeping up with him was a challenge,' Scott says. 'I'm no acrobatic pilot, but I had to learn quickly how to throw the paraglider around if I wanted to participate in the flight with him.'

Scott set up his raptor rescue facility in Pokhara in 2001. People bring wounded birds to the rescue centre and Scott does what he can to rehabilitate them before releasing them back into the wild. Early on, he was brought an Egyptian vulture chick, which he named Kevin. After years of care and intensive training, Kevin became a great 'para-hawking' bird, a term Scott coined one night in a bar. This new branch of the project developed and expanded at the same time as the discovery that vulture populations in Asia were plummeting, leaving some species, including the Egyptian vulture, endangered. In offering flights with Kevin – brief opportunities for people to participate in a bird's world – Scott's aim is that people 're-see' vultures. They are dynamic, graceful and well worth preserving. Conservation and adventure combine.

*

During my first few days in Nepal, I begin to get to know this new place in which I find myself. I spend one morning at the Matepani Gumba Buddhist monastery on the edge of Pokhara, where a young monk offers me a cup of yak-butter tea and lets me sit in on the morning's meditation. When I get up to leave, I am handed a card that wishes me 'a brilliant and prosperous 2068'. Nepal uses the Vikram Samvat calendar, which is 56.7 years ahead of our Gregorian calendar, but it's delightful to be encountering, here, the same dislocating sense of having stepped outside of time that I associate with flying.

I also spend a day with the British Gurkhas, who are based at Pokhara and come to the lake to paraglide. Two instructors, eight Gurkhas and I drive up a steep winding path, then leave the trucks behind to hike through stepped farms, passing haystacks and women bent over working in the fields. As we ascend and the wind gets up, my radiotherapy scar begins to burn, along with my fast-beating heart. We arrive at the launch point, where a green ribbon on a stick acts as a windsock and shows that the wind is coming from the east. A paraglider whistles overhead. When I ask why the military includes paragliding courses in its training, I'm told that it improves the soldiers' capacity to endure fear. At that, I smile.

*

That night, I settle into my hut next to the aviaries and listen to the bells on the anklets of the birds as they jingle with their movements. The soundscape here is a rich mix.

Dogs bark, goats bleat and the generator purrs, filling the
hot air with the scent of diesel. Later, I wake up to hear
rats scrabbling in the straw roof and, beyond them, an
extraordinary storm. The thunder echoes and reverberates
in the mountains to create a sound I've never heard before,
it seems to incorporate the very mountain rock. Even the
dogs fall silent.

Chapter Sixteen

The Rapture of Raptors

On my third morning at Scott's centre, I pick up a copy of the English-language Nepalese newspaper, the *Nepali Times*. On the front page is a cartoon drawing of the Prime Minister of Nepal, Bhattarai, depicted as a hunched black vulture, standing on a pile of human skulls. It is this traditional image of the vulture with its head in a bloody carcass that Scott wants to show me before I can get up in the air with his birds.

Scott's project is funding a 'vulture restaurant' in Gachowk, near Pokhara, but he wants to show me another one, on the edge of Chitwan National Park, half a day's drive to the south-east of Pokhara. This vulture restaurant is based at a cow sanctuary, where cows are kept until they die naturally and can be taken to the clearing on the edge of the jungle to offer vultures a diclofenac-free carcass. The rescue centre is apparently extremely comfortable – one cow has been there for six years.

We park in the village and walk half a mile or so to a large clearing. In one corner, there is a wooden hide on stilts; it reminds me of the witch Baba Jaga's hut on chicken legs in the Russian fairy tale. A dead cow is carried

into the clearing and, as it is laid out, I walk around the
site. A whole perfect black hoof looks like a child's tiny
shoe. Skulls, rib cages, leg bones are strewn everywhere,
dry and white; they crunch underfoot, three-quarters
buried in the grass. I stumble on a vertebra. To my left, a
jawbone juts up out of the green, surrounded by delicate
blue flowers. Death is here in stark and brutal clarity.

We settle into the hide, on hard wooden benches, and
peer out of the thin slit in the wall, as vultures slowly
arrive to descend into the trees on the edge of the clearing. Dhan Bahadur Chaudhary (DB for short), the project
leader, is with us and, as a deer barks in the distance, he
explains it is a warning call from further into the jungle;
a leopard was spotted a few days ago, close to the village.
They come to the feeding site to chew on skeletons, and
there are tigers, rhino and sloth bears here too. I've
already been told what to do if we see any of them: run
from a sloth bear, stand still for a tiger and climb a tree
from a rhino.

Two Egyptian vultures flop on top of a silk-cotton tree.
Five dark, wiry-haired wild boar graze in the distance.
A pair of white-backed vultures perch in a high tree. A
jungle babbler chirrups and a couple of crows perch on an
upturned ribcage, close to the carcass. The morning mist
slowly lifts as the level of heat in the jungle rises. As we
watch, eating our hard-boiled eggs and samosas, more and
more vultures arrive.

'They won't rush on to the carcass,' Scott explains.
'They will spend some time watching, waiting; they are

making certain that the cow is dead and that it's safe to come down.' The holy creature – this humble god – lies on its side, its head resting on the ground. Moth-eaten, bony, stubborn, it should be sitting on some dusty street, but, out here in the jungle, its lifeless body makes for a strangely peaceful sight.

We are cold and restless in the hide. Thoughts stray, we talk, stare into space, momentarily forget about the carcass in front of us. We talk about birds, and Scott admits that he thinks human attitudes to birds are often misplaced, especially when we look at birds as images of freedom.

'Birds soar to save energy,' he points out. 'Birds aren't flying around, enjoying being free.' All birds of prey live on a fine line between hunger and survival because they have no fat reserves to rely upon – they would be too heavy to fly, if they did. They constantly need to stay within a narrow zone where they can balance their nutritional needs with the fitness and lightness that enables them to fly and hunt. So soaring is an aspect of their survival that runs deep, and may be even more powerful and instinctive than hunting for food. It is all driven by the need to conserve energy.

Eerie jungle sounds surround us. Scott says he can hear the cry of a crested serpent eagle. There must be at least fifty vultures now perched in the leafless trees that edge the clearing. At last, one or two descend to the carcass, gliding down to land, and hop along the ground before climbing on top of it. Soon, others follow, until it is covered in a writhing mass of giant birds. There are Himalayan griffon vultures and white-backed vultures, and a steppe eagle. The carcass is invisible beneath a crowd of huge birds bent over the meat, pushing each other, their giant dark-brown wings flapping. Some are standing on the carcass, others leap and shove to get on to it. But the scene is not gruesome; the birds squawk and squabble somewhat, but mostly they get on with eating.

After half an hour or so, some birds come away from the group and stand with their wings half open, their crops full, digesting. As we watch, Scott tilts his head towards me and says, 'A large vulture will gorge as much food as possible when it eats, and sometimes they are so full they are unable to fly away.' Most of the Himalayan griffon vultures brought in to Scott's sanctuary are in fact perfectly healthy, but just fully fed. If they are approached by humans, they will attempt to fly away, but can't, and people wrongly think they are injured. I can see that it would be hard for them to take off.

An hour later, the carcass is no more than a skeleton. Many of the birds have managed to run and take off to land in trees nearby; a few vultures are still at the carcass. All of a sudden, from the left, two golden jackals come charging on to the scene. Vultures leap at them, claws out, hissing; the jackals squeal and bark and stop still, staring at the skeleton. They soon slope off.

*

The following morning, I finally meet Kevin, Scott's Egyptian vulture and the bird he parahawks with. We are driving with Shiva, Scott's neighbour, along a winding road in his old Maruti to the launch point, at Sarangkot, on a hill above the lake. Scott is in the front passenger seat with Kevin perched on his gloved hand, unhooded. Over Scott's shoulder, Kevin peers at me with an amber eye. The fine white feathers circling Kevin's head make him look like a mixture of Ziggy Stardust and Queen Elizabeth I, with her white ruff; there's something both rock and regal about this bird. He looks like he was born old.

At the launch point, a dusty flat top above a 2,000-foot drop down to Pokhara, a Himalayan griffon vulture is flying overhead. Shiva holds Kevin on his left hand and speaks into his mobile phone with the other, while Scott prepares the paraglider.

I am strapped into the harness in front of Scott, given a falconer's glove for my left hand, and asked to wear a pouch around my waist, which is full of chopped buffalo meat. I will feed Kevin in the air. I'm nervous that I will stumble on the take-off, but we stand into wind, the paraglider wing fills with air and we launch smoothly, running down the hill and then lifting off into the open valley below.

Shiva releases Kevin, who flies fast out into the valley ahead of us, soaring at seventy kilometres an hour. All around us are the icy peaks of the Annapurna Range, the rocky triangle of Machhapuchhre moving in and out of view as clouds pass up and around it. Pokhara is in a haze, thousands of feet below, and it's encircled by hills stepped with small fields. The lake is a dark silvery plain beneath us.

I settle into my harness and ferret in the pouch in front of me for a piece of buffalo meat. My palm is sweaty inside the leather falconer's glove. I put a piece of meat between my thumb and forefinger and cover it with my other hand so that the sharp-eyed vulture cannot see it, as Scott has instructed me.

Scott blows his whistle, I thrust my gloved hand out with the buffalo meat on it and Kevin flies in from somewhere behind us. He lands perfectly on my hand, decelerating from seventy kilometres an hour in a matter of seconds. He snatches the meat and then swoops off the gloved hand to the left and is swallowed again in the sky's currents, which have become as thick as water at this speed. Watching this vulture on the ground and then soaring in the sky is the difference between seeing a penguin on ice and then swimming through the ocean. As he shoots beneath and around us, I watch with fascination the micro-movements of his wings and tail feathers adjusting with the air. Compared to his easy agility and grace, we are stiff and awkward, like some lumbering flying bus.

The air is cool and fresh on my face as we push through it, as it rushes all around me. Scott swears in frustration at the sky because he's finding it hard to find lift, even though there are wild birds soaring all around us. A Himalayan griffon vulture flies right beneath me, its speckled brown two-and-a-half-metre wingspan stretching either side of my feet. A wild Egyptian vulture flies below us, too, but further away, so Scott isn't worried that Kevin will be distracted by it. Scott is more comfortable flying with the larger vultures, he says, the Himalayan griffon vulture, white-backed vulture, cinereous and red-headed vultures, as these are friendlier than the Egyptians, even though it is an Egyptian vulture that he has trained to fly with him. 'Flying towards a gaggle of vultures is no problem, or a gaggle of vultures flying towards me,' says Scott. But he is super-wary of wild Egyptian vultures during breeding season, and stops flying altogether if there are Egyptians breeding nearby.

Vultures can follow thermals, convergence lift and wave, Scott explains, because they can see the particles of dust and insects rising up in the disturbed air. Vultures might use free-flight pilots as thermal markers — 'It's nice to think you might be useful' — but Scott acknowledges that it is more likely that the birds have seen a butterfly or other insect being carried higher. They are flying around in a different sky to the one we see; we only see through the air, but it's a moving, visible body to raptors. As Scott describes how his vultures read the sky, I am reimagining it — once again, the sky is transformed for me, and now I'm seeing it in even more detail.

Scott whistles again, I hold out my hand, Kevin swoops in and I see his feathers, tight next to me, ruffling in the wind before he flies off again, speeding into the sky without flapping, working the currents, his wings perfectly in tune with his element. I watch him soaring around us and a little spark ignites inside my chest, sending a jolt through my torso and stomach, a feeling of rapture surging through me.

The word 'raptor' means 'to tear', and refers to any bird with a hooked beak designed for tearing flesh. Soaring with this raptor, I am struck by a feeling of being carried away, connecting to the rapture I experience in the air. Illness has broken me open, made room for this experience, made it possible for me to soar with raptors – to soar like them, even. They have become my guides, but it goes far deeper than that: they are showing me the way to rapture. This upwelling is a splitting open, a tearing. My whole journey into free flight connects to the breaking open caused by breast cancer, the breaching of my borders, my skin – the very edge of myself cut into. My experience of illness was a ripping away from the known world on the ground, but learning to soar is like being carried off. The only way into this rapture was through the rupture. I know I am getting carried away, and yet I can't help it. The rapture of flying is a feeling of taking off, being taken over, overpowered, overwhelmed. I let go into it, and it sizzles up my spine. I am carried aloft in its claws.

Scott lets me take the controls. My gloved hands can hardly fit into the handles of the paraglider, but I work them in and then pull and release so we make an 'S' turn as we fly over the lake. It feels fantastic to take the reins. The bright yellow wing filters golden light on to my face. We wind down over the lake to land on its edge. Scott's landing is highly controlled, but I sit down hard on my bum and the yellow wing collapses on top of me. Kevin has returned to his aviary.

*

A week later, I am about to set off on the long journey back to Wales. As I wait for my taxi, I look up and the dark shape of a Himalayan griffon vulture soars across my view. From here, it looks like it is holding its body perfectly still, the constant micro-movements of each metre-spanning wing invisible to my clumsy human eye. The vulture turns steeply into the wind, slowing down to make the most of the thermal and, as it is lifted, it shrinks in my perspective. I strain to hold it in focus. An eye-drying wind blows across my face. I blink the dust out. I can hear nothing down on the ground, the bird seeming to fly in silence, but I imagine the air loud and rushing up there, vibrating the tiny bones of its inner ear. I'm an unknown grounded darkness down here, possibly a threat to the cautious vulture above me, but I know its eyesight is about twenty times better than mine. I imagine it glancing down briefly, on a turn, perhaps, to look at me staring up, seeing clearly my hand held up to shade my eyes, the gaping hole of my mouth a cave of questions.

As we drive away from Pokhara, heading for a bus that will take me to Kathmandu and the airport, car horns toot, the buildings on the edge of town gradually thin and disappear, and we enter the countryside, dotted with haystacks. I can see the vast, impossibly high icy ridges of the Himalayas more clearly without any buildings in the way. They seem to grow larger as I move away from them.

Chapter Seventeen

Skybound, Earthbound

> '[Bird] Flight thrills us because it suggests the weight-
> lessness we cannot achieve but also the freedom of
> mind that we can.'
>
> Tim Dee

I return to Wales, move back into the chapel, and feel like
something has been exorcized. The flying is good, most
days, and Bo and everyone at the gliding club seem
restored, yet I am restless. Since I was a child, my parents
and I have frequently taken our sleeping bags outdoors for
nights under the open sky. Unprotected, each time I feel
as though I have left something of myself there, and now I
have an urge to sleep outside again, to be gathered to the
ground.

On a clear, moonless evening in June, close to the longest day, I pack a rucksack and head to the gliding club. I
choose a spot in the long grass on the edge of the airfield,
near to the landing strip, and settle into my sleeping bag
and a waterproof bivvy bag. I drift off as the sky is turning
orange, and later wake in the dark, digging myself out of

a deep sleep to see the Milky Way spilt above me, slowly turning and framed by the oval opening around the top of my sleeping bag. I lie still, taking in the space and the silver points of ancient light. With my back to the earth, held tight to the ground, I think of myself as lying at the bottom of the great sphere of the planet, peering down into the universe; the stars are beneath me. I am surrounded by almost total silence.

The next morning, four hares are hopping about on the main landing strip, skinny, brown, with long, strong legs and bulging eyes. They sit and stare at me for a moment, ears flicking at this strange sight. I watch them leaping and preening, chasing each other. Perhaps they slept close by in their own form, while I had slept in mine.

I pack up my things, including water, hard-boiled eggs and the fresh rolls which Bo has brought me, wandering across the airfield to deliver them in their still-warm paper bag. I set off in the middle of the balmy summer day to climb up into the Black Mountains, to the highest peak, Waun Fach, because I know where I need to go and sleep next: I have to return to the burn scar on Pen Trumau.

It is a steep climb up the first ridge and my pack feels heavy against my shoulder, weakened from the radio-therapy. There is a chilly wind blowing up the north-west-facing ridge, and the sky is full of cumulus. Meadow pipits twitter above me, ravens kronk, agile house martins weave in the moving air currents, riding up on the ridge lift before turning and diving back down into it, to catch the insects being blown up the hill.

I stop to catch my breath and, at my feet, I see a scattering of what I assume are sheep bones, though they could be from a fox. Small vertebrae litter the path like a handful of thrown dice. I pick up a bone and turn it over in my hand, sticking my finger through the hole in the middle and marvelling at its intricacy. I drop it again, and glance up to see a buzzard soaring, working the ridge lift; then I see a glider wheeling in a thermal overhead and turn my binoculars on to it, listening as it hisses towards the bowl of Y Das, above my head. I watch the buzzard and the glider, fascinated by both, and yet I am enjoying the feeling of taking my body up the mountain under its own power, the sensation of my heart pulling me upwards. I don't feel the need to be up in the air.

Halfway up the steep incline, at 1,000 feet, I stop to rest, and lean forward with my heavy pack on my back, so my nose presses into the high mossy bank that edges the path. I close my eyes and inhale the musty smell of soil – alive, cool, mulchy – a deep smell of things in the process of both decay and becoming.

Thoughts and memories from these past years – some, painful moments during my treatment – begin to flash in front of me. I try to concentrate on what is here: my leg muscles feeling the weight of my pack, the sound of a flock of crows in the distance, the last remnants of the may blossom, sheep bleating below in the valley. And the sky, always the sky. That is something that has changed. Now, I see it from a glider pilot's point of view, even when on the ground; I cannot help but read and interpret its lift and sink. I've brought some sky literacy back to the ground with me.

I hear a particularly near and loud skylark, and look up to see it is directly in front of the sun, a black flickering shape in the middle of a gold disc. The sounds of the skylark and the wind blur together into a voice I think I can almost understand.

I finally reach the top of the ridge, and look over to the south and to the dark scar on the top of Pen Trumau in the distance. I am nearly there.

As I walk, it is hard to tell if the white fibres I constantly disturb with my boots are sheep wool or cotton grass. I pick up a piece of lost white wool, an inch or so long, which was wrapped around some pale green coral-like lichen, and worry it between my fingers, pulling at its wiry softness as I walk. I can hear so many skylarks, but, when I look up, I can't see a single one. The path is edged with emerald-green star-shape sphagnum moss; I reach down and plunge my fingers into it; it is damp and softly prickly. The wind rushes through the long, spiky, tough grass, so the ground seems to be whispering, and it joins with the faint moan of another glider soaring ahead, out in the valley.

As I reach Pen Trumau and head to the burn patch, the wind is flying up the west-facing ridge on which the scar is located, gnawing away at it. This time, the patch looks to me like a gash in the peat. Twisting gullies have gouged and cut down further through it, revealing white rock; it looks as if the flesh of the hill has been torn open to the bone. Rain has washed the soil downhill, preventing new growth taking root, and though more wool has been pegged into the patch since I last visited, much of it has worn into the peat. Very little is growing here still.

Perhaps it's too early to tell, but the patch doesn't appear to have improved. It's a wound rather than a scar. Scar tissue binds tightly, is strong, but this ground is open and vulnerable. The scar on my chest is healed, the skin stronger than ever and closed off to the world, but I recognize something of the psychological wound of my illness, here. That is still open, and I think I want it to stay that way, because it is through this wounded place that I have found the rapture of flight. A year ago, I couldn't look at this burn patch, because it represented my own scar and my desperation to be healed, to return to things as they were, to begin as if I'd never been cut open. But that was never going to be possible, and I have healed in a different way. The emotional wound of cancer, like the wound on Pen Trumau, is still open. I have let it navigate me, and it has turned my attention skyward.

I set off to look for a sheltered spot to camp. The east-facing side of the ridge is out of the wind, but steep, and it takes some time to locate a place flat enough to sleep on. I drop my pack, staking a temporary claim, get out the gas stove and heat up a can of tomato soup. The ground here smells strongly of sheep. I climb into my sleeping bag and sit looking over towards the Llanbedr valley and the Sugarloaf, sipping my soup.

Here, on the top of the mountain, I am in between sky

and ground, and on the border between England and Wales, not far from Offa's Dyke; I can see into England, and have a view of the Skirrid mountain, which stands almost exactly on the border. I am a borderland character, I think, coherently liminal, culturally between England and Wales, between identities and languages, between Russian, from my dad's mum, and English, in the other part of my make-up. Disbarred from identifying as Welsh, shouldering the awkward status of incomer, I've identified, from the time we moved here, with my local patch, the valley in which the farm is nestled and the hills around it. I've poured myself into the walnut tree at the bottom of the yard, into the ruined cottage at the top of the farm, into the shapes of the fields and into the hollow ash tree at the bottom of the farm.

In other ways I flicker, too; I feel an affinity with the edge. The border is where I am safest, it offers another place I can flee to, if necessary, and it is a creative space to inhabit, where things remain flexible. Here, nothing is hardened or crystallized. Here, I can keep moving along that liminal edge.

I now know I have to get back to the ground to earn a living, but whatever I do next, I will take the lessons from learning to fly back down with me. I will turn towards the turbulence, for there the lift will be; I will accept that I must move through lumpy rotor to get to the smooth wave; I will ride the edges between things, wary of the sink lurking on the other side.

*

I lie down to sleep at nine o'clock, exhausted from the hike up, with my head pointing out of the sleeping bag, looking south-east. I wake in the dark to see a few stars visible beyond the cloud cover. It is completely silent – no wind, no bleating sheep – so utterly quiet that I can hear the rushing electric ocean of white noise inside my own head. I can't recall the last time I experienced such total silence. Suddenly, I hear something – someone calling my name behind me, a woman's voice I don't recognize. But there is no one there. Drifting in and out of sleep, it is as though my brain is disturbed by the silence and is shouting my name just to hear something, an aural hallucination.

*

I wake the next morning when it is already light, about six, and sit up to look out at the horizon. But I can see nothing. The hill is enveloped in cloud, the fog so thick I can only see a few metres in front of me. I have been warned from childhood not to go on to the hill in fog and especially not on my own. I brew coffee on the gas and ready myself to try to get off the mountain. I picture the path I need to take in my mind, the various forks and cairns that will mark my correct route. I can't even tell where the sun is.

As I walk through the fog, everything becomes obscure; the passage of time is hard to tell, as is the distance. I can't tell if I've walked too far along the ridge and missed the path to the left that will take me down, or if I've not walked far enough and am still on the first ridge of the two I need to cross to get to the path.

The various routes I try become a blind labyrinth. I head straight on a small path, certain at last of my direction, then come across a stone that I am sure I saw behind me. I stride along another path, certain it is the main route, only for it to fizzle out into heather. Wrapped in this wraithlike mist, recognizable landmarks become unfamiliar. Did I see that rock, that sheep windbreak, that cairn? Circling a cairn, I become further disorientated, unable to remember which direction I arrived at it from originally. It is tempting to just sit down and wait, wait for this fog to lift, but it could last for days. No one will find me; I have to find myself.

Disorientated and confused, I give up on paths and decide to try and walk straight downhill, to get beneath the clouds. The gentle slope I am descending is soon aggressively steep. I peer down the almost sheer mountainside, the ground slippery and dangerous in my wet boots. I think better of it and climb back up again, trampling across heather and winberries, following narrow sheep trails, increasingly exhausted.

I am beginning to panic. I feel trapped by the cloud, as though the sky is holding me up on the mountain, preventing me from getting down. I decide that all I can do is stick to the first significant path I come across and follow it until it leads me somewhere – I just have to hope it won't be back up the mountain to Waun Fach. Placing my sodden boots along narrow sheep trails, I continue back up the hill, plodding on through the mist.

And then, suddenly, I stumble on a well-trodden path. Slowly, it begins to descend. This must be a way out. It is eerily silent in the mist. The skylarks aren't singing; I can't see a single bird. The sheep are silent too, their white wool blurred into the fog so they aren't visible until I come right upon them. They turn and stare at me, blank eyed, pausing momentarily in their chewing.

The path begins to descend more steeply. I still have no idea where I am, but I don't care; all that matters is that I am going downwards, out of the disorientating grip of the cloud. I look up, just as the clouds thin and part ahead, revealing green fields and hedgerows. I stop and shout with relief, bending over with joyous belly laughter; I am released. The distant fields below open out and there, suddenly, is the airfield in front of me, appearing as out of a magic trick. I am on the very path I have been searching for all along.

I continue to descend and, at about 1,500 feet, I emerge from the cloud altogether. I turn and look back up at the mountain ridge, which disappears into greyness, fog merging into the sky. I feel as though I have surfaced from a strange other world, an Alice-in-Wonderland mountain on which paths shrink and grow and bend back on themselves. I am back. I am down. I am home. Two kites wheel overhead, flapping occasionally to contend with the weak lift.

*

When I first began to fly, I found myself asking questions. Could the sky feel me here? Was it holding me up for some reason? There is something so animate about the atmosphere. But, today, descending from the mountain has felt like a test, the sky holding me against my will and challenging me to find my way back down to the ground. I have passed the test, I have made it down, and now I need to begin again with life on the ground.

Orville Wright said a strange thing when asked what it was like to fly: 'I got more thrill out of flying before I had ever been in the air at all – while lying in bed thinking how exciting it would be to fly.' The question for me is how to keep the wound open without flying, how to bring the lessons from the sky and the opening up to risk and fear back to a life on the ground. I will find a way, and I will continue to fly, like Orville Wright, in my imagination, soaring with birds, the hope with feathers.

Afterword

And here is where Rebecca temporarily ended her book, with a return to Emily Dickinson's poem. She had been struggling with her health for a couple of months, but following medical tests that revealed nothing, with characteristic strength and determination, she went up to Cove Park in Scotland to take up a literature residency she had been awarded. There, she would finish *Skybound*. But her time at Cove Park was cut short by illness, and, when she came home, further blood tests showed that the cancer had returned in her abdomen.

Bec moved back into her childhood room at the farm, and once again we battened down the hatches, and fourteen months of the terrible treatment followed, delivered at the hands of extraordinary doctors and nurses, desperately trying to change destiny. Bec endured it all with peace and calm, using everything that studies in mindfulness and meditation had taught her, with the constant love and support from her wider family and her many, many friends, all over the world, horrified that she was going to have to do this again. Their cards, emails and small gifts brought her lovely smile to her face so often, in spite of her exhaustion. With her openness, honesty and love, she made the whole process as easy for us as she could. She told the specialists that the only reason she continued with the treatment was for those who loved her, and, because of them, she would not give up. Being able to care for her so intimately was a real gift for us, her parents. When the moment came to let her go, we knew that absolutely nothing more could have been done by us or by science. It was time to stop the struggle in spite of our breaking hearts; she needed to rest.

Bec died on Saturday, 17 September 2016, with Tony, Bo and me sitting, chatting round her, as we always did. She leaves all those who knew her run through with rivers of grief, but her legacy is such that she would be pleased. The students she taught continue to write, crediting her with allowing them to find their voice. Where she was working with schoolgirls who struggled with dyslexia, funding has been found to continue the creative writing workshops.

To learn that you flew high
over the landscape, was a surprise.
I wished I'd known when I introduced you to my
        dyslexics who wanted to write,
but had been told they couldn't, write or read!
But they did, after flying with you, write and read
        beautiful and meaningful words,
Given flight
In our library.

(Written at a memorial evening for Rebecca at Arts Alive, in Crickhowell, by John Clarke, himself an aspiring pilot and the teacher in charge of the girls with whom she worked.)

We knew that, underneath her deep, deep grief, Bec felt very loved and cherished. One day, she put her arms round me and said, 'Don't worry, Mum. Whatever happens, it will be all right. Love is the only thing that matters at all in the end.' And she is right, of course, but it will take time to come to terms with the cruel absence of you, my darling daughter, it will take time.

And there is *Skybound*, of course. We promised her that it would be published, and in the months after her death, Bec's editor, Sophie, and I set about sifting through her countless notebooks, determined to make sure that nothing Bec had intended for the book was left aside. One piece surfaced in a file of 'Misc Writings', sent to Bo in New Zealand when she was back home, and we couldn't help wondering if it is where Bec would finally have wanted *Skybound* to close. We will never know, but it is copied below, and I hope it is what she would have wanted. Though we wish she'd been here to see it out in the world, Bec's death doesn't change what *Skybound* is: a story about coming close to death, and learning to live and be joyful again.

TRISHA LONCRAINE,
April 2018

The Hurt Hare's Form

We are lying, quiet, in a hare's form of flattened long grass and tall buttercups, which bend and bow around us in the breeze, waving to themselves. He sleeps, this man whose disappointment in himself stops him from realizing that he is one beautiful piece of this big new sky. Above me, the blue is inescapable; the sun, in June, is closest to the earth now, and breathes hot on my bare neck. Perfect cumulus clouds bump and weave above us, towing along the wind, the ground, this very day with them. Bugs crawl up my arms, across this page, but I do not shoo them away; the tickle of the spider across my wrist is a playful thing to me now. I long to be up in the sky, but miss it less when he is with me, this man with the Scandinavian eyes, because he is of that element, from the north, where the sky is visible so much of the light side of the year, and where, when it's taken away during the dark months, people go mad with cold grief. No matter how broken and scarred I am, when I look up into a blue sky, which I now know I can navigate and keep inside me, I feel repaired, revealed, consoled at least, enlivened, as I jump off the cliff of my own pain again and again, to soar on its gale-force currents and wave back at myself in my broken-hearted healing. We are all broken; we are alright.

1st January

So. Here we are, standing on the other side of that black line drawn in the golden sand. The line that not even the great mythical gods can cross, the border, the acknowledged end of things. I stand and look at it, the in-coming tide making the sand soft, sucking at my boots, pulling me in and down . . .

It is so unfair, so unbelievable, so unjust, so undeserved, so unconsidered – you could not write it in fiction. Nobody could. This pain has no words.

Each time we turn. We have to. We face the empty beach. This is the way forward, hard uphill, a long path we will always move along, against the sucking sand. We have to move away from it, this line of destiny, this terrible truth, with legs aching, lungs heaving, hearts in pieces.

I ponder as I go the unthinkable, undisclosable deals I tried to make with a god who would not listen, with a devil who did not care.

I look back and know that the tide will come in and when it goes back out again, the sea will have claimed it and there will be no line. Surely that is only right, that life will return to how it was. Well, we wait to see, but for now, and for every New Year's Day, it is as it is.

Loved ones come to help, to stand with us, to watch that line, to touch and stroke us, to say and do the right thing when there is no right thing to do or say. 'We know how you feel, we understand,' they say, eyes spaniel-soft and caring, crying to see our pain, helpless against this unyielding, sucking sand. They try to haul us up the beach, but they don't understand that I want to stay. I want to stay in sight of that bleak black line because I don't believe it. I am, still, so sure that it is all untrue, a haunting hurtful nightmare from which I will wake to see her suddenly striding out of that sea, tall, beautiful and well, smiling as she moves toward me, touching me gently with a wet hand, linking her arm in mine as we walk unhindered together up the beach.

That is how it should be. A child, a beautiful child, so loved and cherished – how can this happen to someone so precious as she?

How can this be?

TRISHA LONCRAINE

Glossary

ailerons – long, thin, hinged flaps that stretch across the
    trailing edge of each wing, used to make the glider
    bank.

airframe – the body of an aircraft.

altimeter – the instrument that shows altitude in a glider.

attitude – the angle of a glider's nose against a horizon,
    determining speed.

audio vario – the instrument that shows whether the glider
    is ascending or descending, using a beeping that
    varies in speed and tone.

bunt – a manoeuvre that gives negative G-force in the
    aircraft.

Ceconite – material used to cover the structure of a glider.

chandelle – a steep climbing turn to gain height while
    changing direction.

elevator – situated at the rear of the glider to move the
    nose up and down, controlling speed.

glide ratio – the height a glider descends divided by the
    distance it travels to lose that height, usually
    expressed as fraction such as 1/46 (the glider will
    travel 46 km horizontally while descending 1 km
    vertically).

ground loop – where the tip of one wing hits the ground when moving at speed, spinning the glider around dangerously.

half Cuban – an aerobatic manoeuvre where an aircraft rolls level on the downward side of a loop.

induced drag – an aerodynamic drag force that occurs when a wing creates lift by redirecting the airflow coming at it.

katabatic winds – down-valley evening winds caused by mountain cooling.

land out – to make an emergency landing somewhere other than the airfield.

orographic clouds – clouds caused by wind flow over mountains.

pilot's glory – the shadow of a plane surrounded by a halo of rainbow-like circles.

rotor turbulence – strong turbulence below the smooth wave.

rudder – situated at the rear of the glider, used in unison with the ailerons to control banking in flight.

rudder pedals – two pedals, used by the pilot to control the rudder.

run the wing – to hold and run with one wing tip as the glider moves off the launch point and picks up speed.

stick – situated between the pilot's knees, this controls the elevator and the ailerons.

variometer – instrument to show the glider's rate of climb or descent.

V.N.E. – maximum airspeed of a glider.

Acknowledgements

There are so many people to thank for their support, encouragement and love through the process of both the events that this book describes and the later process of writing the book, that it's hard to know where to begin. So, first, the official stuff: a huge thanks to the Caroline Trust; the Reuben Foundation; the Banff Centre, Canada; Literature Wales and the National Lottery, through the Arts Council of Wales; Cove Park, Scotland; and the Society of Authors, Authors' Foundation.

Thanks to my agent, Jim Gill, for managing so deftly all the aspects of publishing that I don't understand. Enormous thanks to Paul Baggaley at Picador for taking on the project with such enthusiasm and encouragement, and to Sophie Jonathan, my incisive, intelligent and generous editor. And thanks to all the team at Picador for welcoming me to the house so warmly and for believing in *Skybound*.

Deep gratitude to my family, the Lindesays, Powells, Loncraines and Forsters, my grandmothers, Lis Lindesay and Galena Shanley, and Major Stephen Powell, and to friends local and far away; to Joe Griffiths, Polly Beck, Nick Carter, Patience and Alan Rowden, Anne and Cyril Teasdale, Mary and Ivor Parry, Jan and Richard Renshaw, Jane, Madelaine and Mercedes White, Mike and Shelley Stroud, Sally Clare, Roger Sweet, Simon and Nicky Turley, Steve Hesmondhalgh, Jon Mansfield, Harriet Jaine (especially for Kate Bush), Tom and Sally Jaine, Paddy and Liz Hosier, John and Pat Fowler, Peter Allum, Helena Tang, Kate Silk, Matthew Giddings, Tony and Lucy Lindesay, Paul Mew, Kate Lindesay, David and Diana White, Nick and Tan Skeaping, Alison Cobb, Sarah Dustagheer, Jane Griffin, Lawrie Lewis, Sam Lewis, Dani Haywood, Bob and Jenny Lindesay, Richard and Stephanie Horton, Richard and Afreen Saville, Mo and John Moulds, Jane Loncraine, Audrey Tomlin, Helen Lowdell, Andrew Marsham, Farrhat Arshad, Jan Johnson, Deborah Jones, Brontë Flecker, Daria Martin, Olivia Plender, Jake Williams, Stephen Harrington, Carol Morgan, Julia Mines, Shirley Yuval-Yair, Megha-Nancy Buttenheim, Lori Cable and a very special thanks to Ben Brice. A big thanks to writer and editor friends for support and encouragement; to Jack Tackle, John Porter, Lyndsie Bourgon, Aaron Spitzer, Sarah Stewart Johnson, my fellow Mountain and Wilderness writers on the wonderful Banff programme, and the fantastic editors running it with such skill and grace, Anthony Whittome and Marni Jackson, who helped enormously getting the book into shape. Huge thanks to Anthony for ongoing unwavering support after I came home. Thanks also to Niall Griffiths, Jay Griffiths, Paul Henry, Jim Crumley, and to Jim Perrin for pointing out the raptor/rapture connection.

I am very aware that the printed word takes on a certain authority, which, especially in a memoir, is in truth extremely subjective. I know that the story here is my truth, but that many of the same events might have been experienced quite differently by others involved, and their truths are equally valid. So, many thanks to all the amazing pilots I met in Wales, New Zealand and Nepal, who flew with me and shared their stories with me so generously; in particular, in Wales, to John Coward, Keith Richards, Dr Peter Saunby and his grandson Lazlo, Robin Howarth, Don Gosden, Mike Rossiter, Martin Brockington, John Horley, Gerry Martin, Robbie Robertson, Phil Swallow, Dr Emily Shepherd, Sue, Jim, Ben and Joe Harper, Liz Torrence, John Bally, Derek Eckley, and all the members of the Black Mountains Gliding Club, and Julian Brown, Martin Cray and Pete Gallagher. In New Zealand, huge thanks to Gabriel Briffe, G. Dale, Annie Laylee, Lemmy Tanner, Gavin Wrigley, Rod Dew, Ash Hurndell, Philip Plane, Trevor Mollard, Darren Smith, Tony Collins, Trevor Florence, Jenny Wilkinson, Yvonne Loader, Jill McCaw, Terry Delore, Ricco, Justin and Gillian Wills, and Mandy Gerard.

I am enormously grateful for Gavin Wills' generosity in hosting me at Omarama, for offering me such hospitality and friendship, for helping me understand the unique skills of his flying in his beloved Southern Alps, for opening up to me and sharing his experiences with his daughter, Lucy, which helped me so much. I'm eternally grateful for his support.

Particular thanks to Scott Mason, in Nepal, for his hospitality, and for sharing his passion for vultures and conservation, and also thanks to the brilliant wider paragliding community I met in Pokhara, who are now doing such great